I will fight cancer
until my last breath.

−Dick Vitale

ISBN: 978-1-957351-57-5 (Paperback)
ISBN: 978-1-957351-45-2 (Hardcover)

Published by Nico 11 Publishing & Design | Mukwonago, Wisconsin
Michael Nicloy, Publisher | www.nico11publishing.com
Quantity order requests may be emailed to: mike@nico11publishing.com

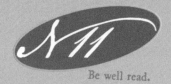

Be well read.

Until My Last Breath: Fighting Cancer With My Young Heroes
Author: Dick Vitale
Contributing Author: Scott Gleeson
Contributing Editor: Erik Brady
Foreword: Mike Krzyzewski
Prologue: Shane Jacobson
Afterword: Scott Gleeson
Mic Drop: Kevin Negandhi
Epilogue: Lorraine Vitale
Proofreader: Lyda Rose Haerle
Interior and Cover Layout: Griffin Mill
Front Cover Image: Harry Sayers
Cover Design: Michael Nicloy

All included images are used by permission of the owners.

Photo credits include the V Foundation, Harry Sayers, the Vitale family, ESPN, and each of the families featured in this book and any promotion associated with it.

Special thanks to Cade Kulak at Mary Kenealy Events for assistance with the gala photos.

Hardcover Printed in Canada | Paperback Printed in The United States of America

All proceeds from the sales of this book are donated to
the V Foundation, Dick Vitale Pediatric Cancer Research Fund

To donate, visit <u>donate.v.org</u>

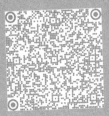

Don't Give Up…Don't <u>Ever</u> Give Up.®

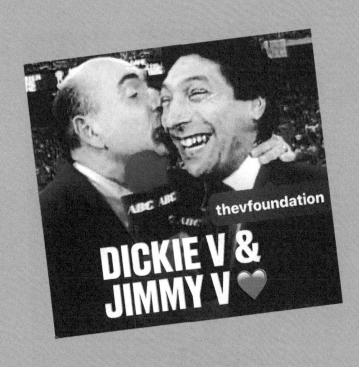

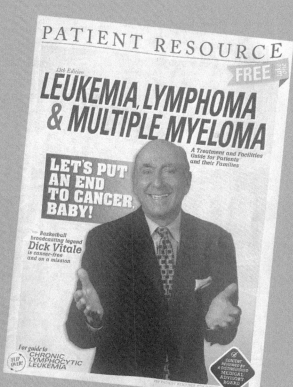

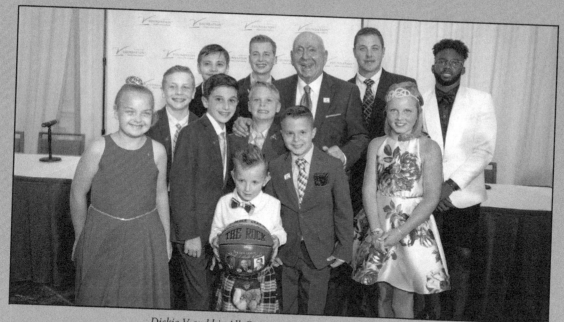

Dickie V and his All-Courageous Team at the 2019 Gala.

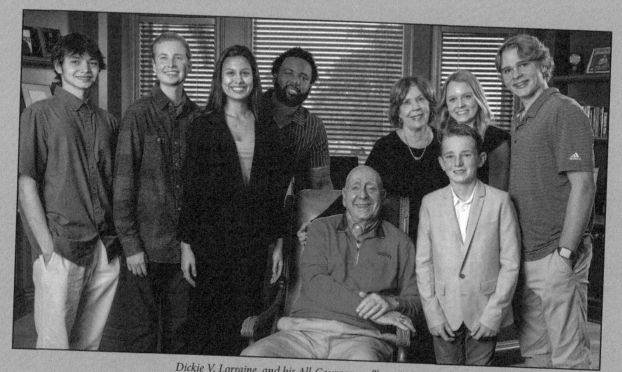

Dickie V, Lorraine, and his All-Courageous Team in 2024.

"Dick Vitale has been an ardent supporter of Jim's vision for the V Foundation since the day we began, and his passion is evident in everything he does. It's been an honor to stand alongside him for the last three decades in the fight against pediatric cancer, and we've made incredible strides toward research and cures for children because of his tireless dedication to a cause that matters to so many families."

– Pam Valvano Strasser

CALLIN' IT FOR DICKIE V AND HIS GALA!

Jay Bilas, ESPN analyst and author of Toughness: Developing True Strength On and Off the Court: "It's hard to imagine college basketball without Dick Vitale because he's embedded into the fabric of the game. He's been the soundtrack to college basketball for so long. But what he means to cancer fighters everywhere will live on forever. By sharing his story publicly, he's given the masses comfort and solace all while he's been going through hell in his own fight. By bringing everybody in, he's expertly illuminating that cancer is not something any of us should have to go through alone."

Jon Cooper, Tampa Bay Lightning Head Coach: "When you see how these All-Courageous kids look at Dick, that right there says it all. They adore him in every way. For these kids to go out of their way when Dick was going through his own cancer battle and try to make him feel better, that comes from all the love he's given them. That relationship he has with them, at 84, is something special and goes beyond basketball or broadcasting. It goes beyond sports."

Jay Wright, Former Villanova Men's Basketball Coach: "To see Dick face a disease he's sworn to fight against for children has been shocking. But how he's handling it – fighting it with passion and putting the kids out front – that's less surprising. Because it's who Dick Vitale is, he's a coach to us all at heart. I'm just in awe of his courage and inspiration."

Fran McCaffery, Iowa Men's Basketball Coach: "With Dick's annual cancer galas, he's unified our coaching community in our fundraising efforts. That's not just pro and college coaches, what he does spreads to high school coaches and young people. His voice in this fight trickles down. We all trust in him to guide the way. When he's no longer with us, no one on this earth will be able to carry the torch at fighting cancer the way he has and approach it with the same intensity and tenacity. No one."

Scott Drew: Baylor Men's Basketball Coach: "There are only a handful of people who have done more for college basketball than Dick Vitale. The attention, passion and excitement he has brought to our sport are unmatched and every one of us involved in this sport are indebted to him for his contributions. Maybe even more impressive, though, is how Dick has used this platform God has given him to bring awareness, raise money and join the fight against pediatric cancer. While fighting his own battle with cancer, Dickie V has been unwavering in his mission to fund research and save as many lives as possible, leading the charge to put an end to this terrible disease. He is an amazing human being who has made this world a better place."

Rick Pitino, St. John's Men's Basketball Coach: "I've been coaching for 48 years and known Dick since he was a high school coach. There are so many people who have protected our game but none more than Dick. He's the face of college basketball and one of the main reasons our sport has stayed as popular as it has. But, his legacy will be about what he's doing for people. I lost a son so when Dick fights for children who come down with cancer, it is very dear to my heart. Children suffering is the worst feeling in the world. Dick hasn't been afraid to join the fight, even with his own struggles, and that's remarkable."

John Calipari, Kentucky Men's Basketball Coach: "Dick is a builder, not a demolisher. And for what he's built, we should build a statue of Dick Vitale to repay him. His legacy in my mind will be that he's always used his platform to add value and help other people. What he's done for basketball – impacting millions – and what he's done for coaches especially is immeasurable. He's 84 and he asks himself, 'who am I going to help today?' His tombstone will read: He used his life and his fame to help children. What's better than that?"

Bill Self, Kansas Men's Basketball Coach: "I'd like to give a shout out to Dickie V for the courageous efforts he has put into fighting his own cancer and certainly the role he's played in raising money specifically for pediatric cancer through the V Foundation. He's done a lot of things to help so many through the media and through basketball, but what he's done off the court far surpasses anything he's done on the court."

Rick Barnes, Tennessee Men's Basketball Coach: "I think God has used Dick in a powerful way in how he becomes deeply affected by these kids on his All-Courageous Team. When one of them hurts, a piece of him hurts with them. This whole time he's been going through cancer himself, he never stopped doing what he set out to do – raise money for pediatric cancer until his last day."

Roy Williams, former North Carolina Men's Basketball Coach: "Dick is the greatest of all the ambassadors for college basketball. He loves the game, its players, coaches and officials, and also the fans. His passion for our sport is unmatched. I have even greater admiration for the relentless energy he has given towards raising so much money to fighting cancer, particularly pediatric cancer. It's just phenomenal. Anyone who reads his book will find themselves laughing and crying – it's what he makes you do and he does it very well."

Jim Boeheim, former Syracuse Men's Basketball Coach: "Dick continues to be perhaps the greatest college basketball ambassador the game has ever had. He's been a positive and enthusiastic voice for decades. He's also been a tireless fighter against cancer, from his work with the V Foundation and his specific fundraising for pediatric cancer research. Dick's recent personal battle against cancer has been a real inspiration."

Tom Izzo, Michigan State Men's Basketball Coach: "I've had the honor of attending Dick's gala and the stories from the families who have children battling forms of cancer are emotional and heartbreaking. Standing beside all of those families is Dick, who has made it his mission to raise as much money as he can in the fight against pediatric cancer. His own personal courageous battle against vocal cancer has just made him work even harder. Dick has fought like hell in his own battle and there is no doubt in my mind that he will continue to fight for young kids and their families because there is no quit in him."

Mike Woodson, Indiana Men's Basketball Coach: "Dick Vitale has given so much to the game of basketball as a coach and broadcaster, but his three victories over cancer are the greatest of his career. The most important work of his Hall of Fame career is his commitment to defeating this awful disease. Dick's dedication to cancer research and funding is extraordinary, and his passion has lifted the spirits of so many. We are all grateful to Dick for his work on and off the court, and he is an inspiration for all of us."

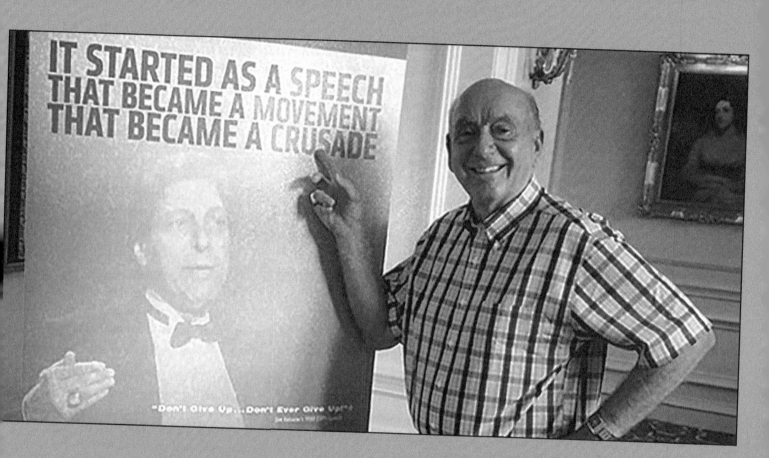

Until My Last Breath

Fighting Cancer With My Young Heroes

By Dick Vitale
with Scott Gleeson

Table of Contents

Foreword with Mike Krzyzewski, Former Duke Men's Basketball Coach   1

Prologue with Shane Jacobson, V Foundation CEO   5

Chapter One – My Fourth Quarter with Jim Valvano & Tony Colton. Dick takes the baton   9
from Jimmy V and makes a deathbed promise to 17-year-old Tony to fight childhood cancers –
until his last breath.

Chapter Two – I Won't Be Silenced with the Dick Vitale Family. Dick loses his speaking voice   17
for four months to vocal-cord cancer, but never stops speaking up on behalf of children suffering.

Chapter Three – Unbeatable Positivity with the Payton Wright Family. Dick highlights the   25
legacy that 5-year-old Payton leaves behind, and how she inspired him to start his unyielding
effort in raising money for pediatric cancer – the genesis for his annual galas.

Chapter Four – Defeating Relapse with the Weston Hermann Family. Dick visits with four-   35
time brain cancer survivor Weston, 17, who finds respite on the ice as a budding hockey star.
Tampa Bay Lightning coach Jon Cooper cameos.

Chapter Five – You're Not Alone with the Sadie Keller Family. Dick spends time with Sadie,   43
16, who was 8 when she launched a viral video series for kids like her battling cancer. Now she
speaks on Capitol Hill to raise awareness for her cause.

Chapter Six – Suffering for a Purpose with the Cole Eicher Family. Cole, 12 when diagnosed   51
with brain cancer, teaches Dick that the "new normal" derived from a cancer fight can offer
profound perspective.

Chapter Seven – Tears of Strength with the Cannon Wiggins Family. Cannon bravely fought   59
Stage IV High Risk Neuroblastoma as a toddler after being diagnosed at age 2. The 12-year-old
beat the odds, but Dick realizes the tragedy behind the decisions parents are forced to make.

Chapter Eight – Post-Traumatic Resurgence with the Enzo Grande Family. Enzo was three   67
when diagnosed with leukemia and saw his family move five times in three years to find the
right treatments. The 16-year-old helps Dick understand how past trauma often intrudes on the
present.

Chapter Nine – Bonded for Life with the Katelyne Ballesteros Family. Katelyne received the   73
gift of life from her brother, Luis, with a timely bone-marrow transplant that helped her defeat
acute leukemia at age 12.

Chapter Ten – Overcoming Depression with the Coleton Korney Family. Coleton, diagnosed   81
with Ewing's Sarcoma at age 12, helps Dick gain a better understanding of how depression and
isolation play a major part in cancer fights.

Chapter Eleven – Discovering Your Inner Voice with the Mikari Tarpley Family. Mikari was   89
diagnosed with Hodgkin's Lymphoma at 15 – a week into the pandemic. The singer-actor-dancer
shows Dick how a cancer fight can ignite your voice.

Chapter Twelve – Unrelenting Faith with the Joshua Fisher Family. Josh's family believes the   97
power of prayer got them through his fight with leukemia, which included 1,200 chemo doses
over 3 ½ years – starting at age 2.

Chapter Thirteen – A Team of Superheroes. Dick introduces us to the mainstays of his All-   105
Courageous Team — and tells us how they uplifted him in his hour of need. With Jared Rascio,
Jake Taraska, Kyle Peters, Tatum Parker, Harper Harrell, Jayden Spencer, Kinsley Peacock, Joel
McConkey, Emily Ayers, Sydney Hassenbein and Lindsey Rose Belcher.

Chapter Fourteen – Hope as Lifeblood with the Austin Schroeder and N'Jhari Jackson   119
Families. Dick explores the cancer experiences of two families: One who lost their son, and
another who still has theirs. Both showcase how providing the contagious gift of hope can be an
antidote to cancer's devastation.

Chapter Fifteen – Family Over Cancer with the Dick Vitale Family. Dick shares how he faced   131
his own cancers with the loving support of his wife, Lorraine, and their daughters, Terri and
Sherri. Rick Barnes, John Calipari, Rick Pitino and Jay Wright cameo from the college basketball
world, as Dick shows his relentless willpower to stay unretired in his broadcasting career.

Chapter Sixteen – My Home Team with Sydney Sforzo, Ryan Sforzo, Connor Krug, Jake Krug   145
and Ava Krug. Dick was always "coach" of the family, but his five grandchildren turn the tables
and coach him up during his cancer battles.

Outro – A Firestorm Against Cancer. Dick once coached the Titans of the University of Detroit.   155
Now he is in a titanic struggle to wipe out all childhood cancers. After ringing the bell to be
cancer free a third time, he is now as reinvigorated as ever to fight alongside cancer-affected
families.

Epilogue with Lorraine Vitale   159

Mic Drop with Kevin Negandhi   163

Afterword with Scott Gleeson   169

In Tribute   173

Acknowledgments   175

About the Authors   177

Foreword

By Mike Krzyzewski

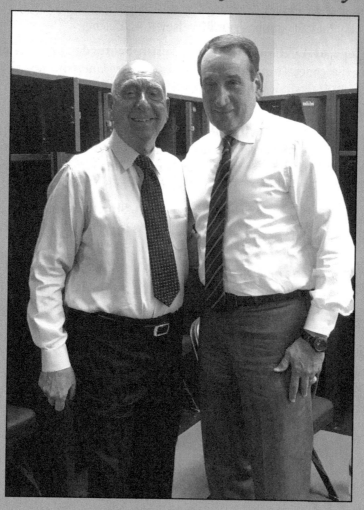

Tireless advocate. Unparalleled supporter. Force multiplier.

In a few words, they describe my dear friend, Dick Vitale. As a former coach and Hall of Fame broadcaster, Dick's impact on the sport of basketball is immeasurable. And although he's not a player, Dick's statistics are, in a couple words, "Awesome Baby!"

- In May of 2024, the Annual Dick Vitale Gala, benefiting pediatric cancer research funded by the V Foundation, will be held for the 19th time.

- Since it started, the Gala, held in Sarasota each year, has raised more than $68 million while becoming one of America's most prolific fundraising events.

- Along with the children who are the event's true MVPs, Dick has celebrated sports legends such as John McEnroe, Patrick McEnroe, Rick Pitino, David Robinson, Jim Boeheim, Alex Rodriguez, and Buster Posey. Derek Jeter, Jeff Gordon, and Jim Kelly will be among future honorees.

- And the best statistic of all – as a result of tremendous efforts across the country such as the Gala, the five-year relative survival rate for childhood and adolescent cancers combined increased from 58 percent during the 1970s to 85 percent among children (during 2011-2017) and 68 percent to 86 percent among adolescents.

Cancer research works!

There have been very few people in my life who've shown as much enthusiasm for the sport of college basketball than Dick. As the former Duke men's basketball coach, I enjoyed countless interactions with Dick over the years as he was preparing for a broadcast, and every time, he made me even more excited about the game I was about to coach. The lens through which he views the world is so optimistic, so upbeat, and so darn pure. For me, those conversations served as a tremendous reminder of why we love college basketball. He showed the entire country HOW we can all have great passion doing so.

In the 1980s, Duke's success coincided directly with the stratospheric rise of ESPN. Therefore, Dick called many of our marquee games back then and for the decades that followed. Let's just say we crossed paths frequently. Our professional relationship grew over the years into a deeply personal one. While we both had our respective jobs to do, Dick and I became great friends who care deeply about one another. As major life events inevitably occurred, we were there for one another. If we were fortunate enough to be in the same room together, hugs and laughter were sure to follow. At other times, we might find ourselves on a lengthy phone call or exchanging text messages.

Early in our relationship, aside from our feelings about basketball, we found we had an even stronger bond in our love for our dear friend Jimmy Valvano, who delivered perhaps the greatest speech in sports history at the ESPYs on March 4, 1993. Dick and I were both with him that night, and we would remain by his side until the very end of his life, when he pledged to never let cancer "win." Jimmy's initial vision and what followed was unimaginable at the time.

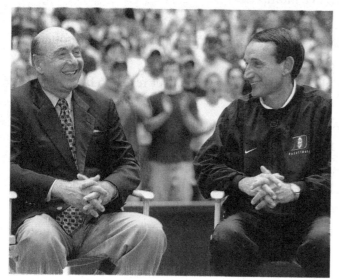

Dick and Coach K in their heyday.

By creating his foundation, Jimmy's legacy outside of basketball would become even larger than the sizable one he established in it.

No one has worked more steadfastly than Dick to raise the necessary funds to help the V Foundation act upon Jimmy's lofty dream to combat cancer. Selflessly, Dick has used his immense popularity and platform to help others, particularly children battling cancer, in such a significant way. He continued to do so while fighting this dreaded disease himself. Though he was impacted directly by the disease he works so hard to defeat, Dick forged through his own share of health challenges, always keeping his efforts to help children at the forefront of his mind.

This led to another book project featuring 16 beautifully presented chapters by Dick and the outstanding writer Scott Gleeson that shares the moving stories of courageous people and their families. Dick's commitment to this "kids first" agenda is as noble as it is unwavering. His diligence over the years changed lives.

Perhaps the best compliment you could pay forward to others would be to read the book with the same emotion and the same love that Dick has exhibited for these children throughout the entirety of his legendary career. His huge heart comes through on every page. The heart, character and strength of these praiseworthy young heroes and their remarkable families will shine even more. Please enjoy.

To donate to the V Foundation,
Dick Vitale Pediatric Cancer Research Fund,
please scan this code.

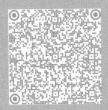

Prologue

By Shane Jacobson
V Foundation CEO

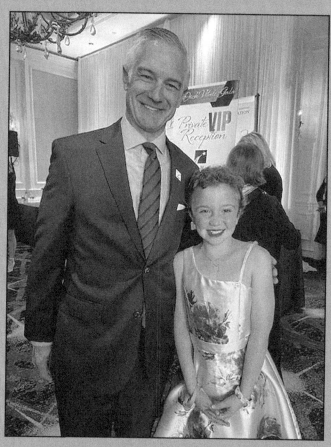

Dick Vitale loves the game of basketball. His passion for the game radiates through the airwaves while he calls games on ESPN. It's something fans never forget.

In the early 1990s, Dick was paired with a well-known, fast-talking, NCAA title-winning coach named Jim Valvano. As a broadcasting duo, their style was electric, feeding off each other's knowledge to create a memorable watching experience.

Thus, the Killer Vees, and their friendship, were born.

A few years later, in March 1993, Jim was set to receive the *Arthur Ashe Courage and Humanitarian Award* at the inaugural ESPYs Awards Show for his perseverance during his battle with cancer. He was sick, very sick, and his family and friends around him were worried that he would not be able to get to New York City for the show, let alone climb the stairs onto the stage and deliver a speech to the world. But Jim was determined.

When the award was announced, Dick met Jim at his seat with a hug and helped him to the podium. Jim delivered an iconic speech in that moment that has inspired millions. His words outlined his "Don't Give Up . . . Don't Ever Give Up!"® spirit, the need for cancer research and the launch of the V Foundation for Cancer Research.

In the final months of his life, Jim quickly built his dream team, a board of directors for the Foundation. He also enlisted his friends to help build awareness for cancer research. Dick has been with us at the V Foundation since the very beginning. And, not surprisingly to anyone who knows Dick – his commitment to us has exceeded 100 percent.

One of the greatest privileges in my role as CEO of the V Foundation is getting to know Dick and Lorraine and seeing their unmatched passion for pediatric cancer research. It is real. They wholeheartedly believe in the power of cancer research to save kids' lives. As a board member of the V Foundation, Dick saw early on what so many children endured when faced with cancer. The Vitales believed change was possible, and there was work to be done.

More than 15,000 children and adolescents are diagnosed with cancer in the United States each year and, sadly, more than 1,500 will die of the disease. These are our children, grandchildren, brothers, sisters, nephews, nieces and friends. As Dick has said many times, no child should ever have to deal with cancer. No parents should ever have to hear the dreaded words, "Your child has cancer."

Children diagnosed with cancer face unique obstacles. Treatment plans can be extremely harsh, as many treatments were designed for adults and not intended for children. This can lead to lifelong effects from treatments, effects that should not inhibit the lives of pediatric cancer survivors. Historically, the support for research has been lacking, with approximately just 8 percent of the National Cancer Institute budget dedicated to pediatric cancer research.

Dick and Lorraine, the V Foundation, and many others are frustrated by the pace of progress and are choosing to do something about it. Dick has championed pediatric cancer research to save lives, using his platform and being a voice for the voiceless. He's quick to post on social media with a statement of encouragement or a plea for help. He sends uncountable text messages every day to inspire people to support the cause. With ESPN, Dick shares his passion on air and rallies others to donate to pediatric cancer research. Because of him, millions have learned of the work being done and seen the power of research into childhood cancers. In 2022, Dick accepted the *Jimmy V Award for Perseverance* at the ESPYS, recognizing his profound contributions to honoring Jim's legacy.

Every year, Dick hosts the Dick Vitale Gala in Sarasota, Florida. It's a collaboration of honored guests from the sports world, featured scientists from the cancer research community, and impactful donors. The weekend is truly one of my favorite weekends of the year. In 2023 alone, the 18th annual Dick Vitale Gala celebrated raising an amazing $12.4 million for pediatric cancer research. Every one of these dollars holds the potential to unlock needed cures and new knowledge about the basic biology of cancer.

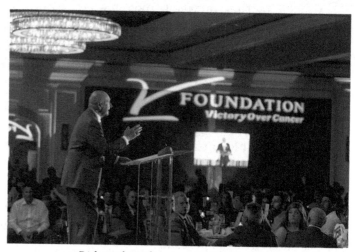

Dick speaks to the crowd at his annual gala.

The meaningful funds Dick raises for pediatric cancer research are put to the best use. At the V Foundation, the Dick Vitale Pediatric Cancer Research Fund has granted more than $84 million to the best and brightest researchers nationwide. Their work is aimed at improving treatment options and saving precious lives, giving kids the opportunities for future birthdays, graduations and weddings – as well as having children of their own. Private funding from organizations like the V Foundation is critical to fill the national funding gap and to advance the novel ideas often imagined by our nation's up-and-coming research scientists.

The good news is cancer research is saving lives today. In the mid-1970s, the five-year survival rate for children was 58 percent. Today, it's 85 percent. We are making a difference, and the research is working. This would not be possible without significant investments from donors and ambassadors, like Dick.

One of the unique and special things Dick has done in support of young cancer patients is forming the Dick Vitale All-Courageous Team. Each year, Dick invites pediatric cancer thrivers to the Dick Vitale Gala to be honored as members of his All-Courageous Team. This provides a front-row seat to an impactful weekend and reminds us how important it is to celebrate progress.

Dick, a Hall of Famer, is a hero to many, but to Dick, the members of the All-Courageous Team and all pediatric cancer survivors are the true heroes, the true Hall of Famers. He puts them first throughout the year and their inspiring stories are what keep him going (and us too). This book provides an incredible chance to meet them, witness how they have become advocates for cancer research (raising money on their own), and see how meaningful lives are saved because of their influence.

The stories you are about to read are their stories. Stories of hardship. Stories of difficult treatment options. Stories of young, innocent lives being impacted by this dreadful disease. But they are stories of fighting. Stories of courage. Stories of never giving up. Stories of benefits from medical advancements only possible because of investments in cancer research.

To those reading this, thank you. Thank you for reading about Dick's work as a hero, a true "prime-time player" for pediatric cancer research, but also the stories of pediatric cancer thrivers, because they are the real inspiration. Proceeds from this book are going to the V Foundation to fund even more cancer research, and for that we are very thankful. Every dollar counts because it could be the next dollar that saves someone you love.

Let me share an example with you. Through the Dick Vitale Pediatric Cancer Research Fund, the V Foundation is currently funding a research project at The Children's Hospital of Los Angeles focused on immunotherapy to treat neuroblastoma, a harsh cancer that affects the nervous system. The project combines chemotherapy and immunotherapy in children who are not responding to chemotherapy alone.

As a result of this work, for half of the children treated in this study, their tumors are melting away. This study shows great progress and would not be possible without funding from the V Foundation and specifically Dick's efforts for pediatric cancer.

Each gift donated to the Dick Vitale Pediatric Cancer Research Fund goes directly to revolutionary pediatric cancer researchers and game-changing projects – 100 percent of it. We are learning new information daily, and with this information we are aiming to improve the lives of children and families faced with cancer. Each discovery brings us closer to victory in the future.

Cancer research done in the past is helping cancer patients today. Because of an incredible team – Dick and Lorraine Vitale, donors, board members, partners and researchers – Victory Over Cancer® is possible. Investments in research today are leading us to tomorrow's victory.

Thank you for teaming up with us in support of pediatric cancer research. Thank you for being part of the V Foundation Team – where our Captain Dick Vitale is leading the way.

To donate to the V Foundation, Dick Vitale Pediatric Cancer Research Fund, please scan this code.

Chapter One
My Fourth Quarter
with Jim Valvano and Tony Colton

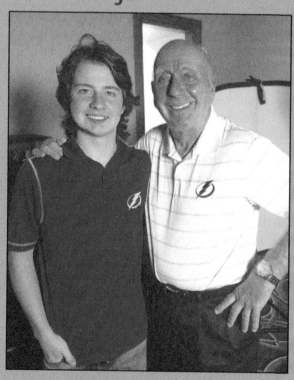

> *"I'm begging you. It may not save my life,*
> *but it could save so many other kids.*
> *Don't let them suffer."*
> *- Tony Colton*

Obsessed.

That's the best word I can use to describe what I feel about raising money for pediatric cancer, fighting for better research to give the oncologists a stronger chance so kids can live another day.

People who know me on the outside probably know me for my famous catchphrases in my four decades-and-counting of calling college basketball games for ESPN. *It's Awesome, Baby*! *Diaper Dandy*! *Dipsy Doo Dunkaroo*!

But those who know me on the inside – on a more personal level – they know my passion for hoops comes in a faraway second place to my true life purpose. That gold medal belongs to fighting alongside the most courageous kids I know. There's no All-American, PTPer or All-Star team that can compete with their heart, their willpower. Trust me on this.

I've gone toe to toe with cancer three times now, first with melanoma in 2021 and then shortly thereafter with lymphoma in 2021 into 2022. After being cancer-free for 14 months, I was diagnosed a third time with vocal-cord cancer.

> *"Think positive and have faith."*
> *- Dick Vitale*

Easily the worst part has been temporarily losing my voice in the winter of 2022 and then again in the summer and fall of 2023. That's because being voiceless took away my ability to fight for all the cancer-stricken kids in the way I know best.

But let me tell you, my friends, cancer doesn't know who it's messing with. I won't be silenced.

Throughout this book, you'll read about my own battles with cancer and the trials I faced. You'll read about the amazing support of my family and how some of the best doctors and nurses in the world helped pull me through.

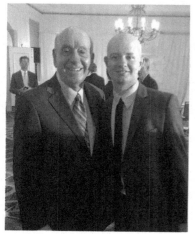

Tony with Dick at his gala.

But the real emotional defibrillator during my own cancer fight each time has come from these kids. I fight for them every single day. They're the players and I'm blessed to be their coach. Make no mistake, though: They're the headliners. If my enthusiasm is at a 10 during March Madness games, consider it at a 20 for what I'm here to share with you in this book.

I want to start by telling you the story of Tony Colton, an up-and-coming teenager who for six years battled clear cell sarcoma of the kidney, a rare and aggressive form of cancer that spread to other areas of his body and prompted over a dozen major surgeries. He battled cancer gallantly, never letting his circumstances overshadow his love for life. He always put others first and had a smile on his face whenever I saw him. Always.

I was at a spring training baseball game in 2017. Tony was 17 at the time. I realized Tony had been presenting himself to me with his armor on most of the time before this. But that day, for a brief second, he took it off. He said to me, "Mr. V, to be completely honest with you, I just got bad news. The cancer's spread all over now." The prognosis was terminal.

I couldn't believe it. Not only because of what he just told me. But because he was smiling the second before, like he hadn't heard the worst news of his life. I asked Tony to come to my annual gala that year and he did, despite the fact that he was dying. He sat at a table with Tampa Bay Lightning coach Jon Cooper and several players – who all adored him. The next day after the gala, during a gathering at my house, Tony asked me if he could speak to the crowd. I told him absolutely.

After humbly standing behind several other cancer survivors, he walked up to the front with a smile on his face and then he took his armor off again – for all of us to see. He said in his impromptu speech, "Listen to Coach V and what he's telling you about raising money for us. Please, I'm begging you. It may not save my life, but it could save so many other kids. Don't let them suffer. I've gone through hell. I'm not here speaking to you asking you for sympathy, but I just want to tell you the truth."

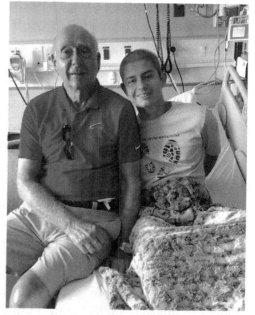

Dick visiting Tony at the hospital.

There was not a dry eye at the house. I'm teary-eyed now just thinking about what he said to everyone about making a difference.

He's so right. The National Cancer Institute – the government agency that is responsible for research and education – received a $6.44 billion budget in 2020. Only four percent of that NCI budget was directed to pediatric cancer (it's since been raised to eight percent).

Are you kidding me? That statistic needs to keep improving not just to save lives, but so that kids can have their own form of treatment instead of putting their bodies through grueling procedures and using medicines created for adults.

It was two months later that I got a call telling me Tony had been rushed to Johns Hopkins All Children's Hospital in St. Petersburg, Florida. Lorraine and I went there to visit him immediately. When we got there, he called me over to his bedside. His voice was raspy, and he could barely talk. He had all these tubes sticking out of him. But he had me come close and said, "Keep doing what you're doing, Mr. V. Don't let others go through what I'm going through. Don't stop raising money for those kids who need help."

That shot me straight through the heart. I mean, think about that. He's dying and all he's doing is thinking about other kids besides himself. I told him, as forcefully as I could, "Tony, I'm going to promise you: Until my last breath, I'm going to beg, plead, do everything I possibly can to raise money to help kids like you. I won't stop."

Tony died at 17, before his senior year of high school. You better believe I'm going to keep that promise I made him. I will fight for kids like Tony until my last dying breath. I remind people often that about 200 Moms and Dads weekly have to hear four words no parent ever wants to hear.

Your child has cancer.

The emotions that parents and kids have to go through are almost too much to bear. I've been involved in a lot of public speaking over the years from banquets to major sporting events. But calling the Final Four internationally doesn't compare to speaking to a mourning crowd after a child has died from cancer. I've spoken at three funerals and I refuse to do it anymore. I just can't take having to see a mother and father put their child to rest again. It tears up my insides.

FACT:
Close to 200 Moms and Dads weekly have to hear their child under the age of 15 has cancer.
-The American Cancer Society

When I was initially told I had bile-duct cancer, in the summer of 2021, I started thinking about my own mortality – like, "the party's about to be over." It was devastating news. I was thinking about not being able to see my grandchildren grow older. I truly feel for all the cancer patients around the world who have to think about that. The emotions just drain your spirit.

That emotional drainage – the same kind I felt at times during my cancer battles these last three years, and the same kind Tony was feeling the day he passed – brings me back to a night I'll never forget, a night many will never forget. That's when my main man, Jimmy Valvano, gave one of the most legendary speeches ever heard in accepting the *Arthur Ashe Courage Award* at the inaugural 1993 ESPYs. Mike Krzyzewski and I to this day talk about how inspired we were because of what we saw behind the curtains, before he ever gave the speech.

Many people were not aware of how much of a struggle it was to even get Jimmy V to New York City for the event. I went to the rehearsal with Joe Theismann the night before and could see how big the night ahead of us at Madison Square Garden was going to be. I called Jimmy to tell him. He was basically whispering on the phone about how he was in such terrific pain and really was only thinking about his family. I never heard him so down. He said to me, "Dick, you think I care about a stupid award? I'm never going to see my daughters (Nicole, Jamie and LeeAnn) grow older. It's over for me." I tried to pick his spirits up, but he wasn't having it.

On the plane, Coach K and his wife, Mickie, were with Jimmy and his wife, Pam. He was puking all over the place on the plane and Coach K said to me, "How is he going to give a speech like this?"

At the arena, I grabbed one of the production assistants. I asked if we could make it easier on Jimmy so he didn't have to walk up there for his speech. Jimmy grabbed me and gave me some choice words, basically saying, "Dick, get me up on that (expletive) stage."

Coach K, Joe Theismann, and I carried him onto that stage. I was mesmerized by his energy when he delivered his speech. He was lifeless on the phone 24 hours earlier and puking on the plane only hours earlier. And then he delivered the speech that to this day serves as a rallying cry for cancer battlers everywhere: "Don't Give Up . . . Don't Ever Give Up!®"

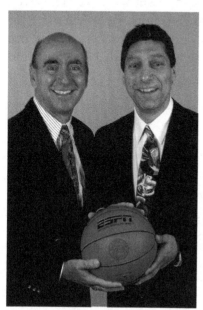

Dickie V and Jimmy V.
(Courtesy of ESPN)

The V Foundation has now raised more than $353 million in his name. His words in that moment play a major role in helping so many people forever in living productive lives because of the research done to honor him. Now that is some kind of legacy to have – one that outweighs the Cinderella national championship that his North Carolina State Wolfpack won in 1983.

I was privileged to call him a dear friend from our time working together as analysts at ESPN. In a way, I feel like he passed me a baton in a relay race to carry on his legacy. I'm a board member for the V Foundation and throw my annual galas in Sarasota, Florida, that have now raised more than $84 million towards pediatric cancer research. That includes more than $17 million in 2023.

I spoke to Jimmy up in heaven at my 2022 ESPYs speech accepting the *Jimmy V Award for Perseverance*. Looking up, I told him, "We're not ever going to stop chasing your dream." Jimmy's dream was to beat cancer. And we're gonna do it.

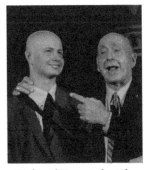

Because the reality is, cancer doesn't discriminate. It doesn't matter your race, religion, or even your age with these kids who have to battle it. Cancer is the ultimate nemesis as an opponent and will bring you to your knees. I know it brought me to mine three times over.

I remember thinking after each major diagnosis: "This disease I've dedicated my life to defeating for kids, I'm battling it now, too." I got so many inspiring messages from all of the courageous cancer fighters who I have relationships with during my battles. I had several kids who have been through what seems like

Dick and Tony at the gala.

thousands of rounds of chemotherapy who told me, "We gotta go see Dickie V and make sure he's alright." If that doesn't tell you how blessed I am, I don't know what does.

The cancer treatments I faced were fricking brutal and had me praying non-stop to St. Jude, the patron saint of hope in troubled times. During those early parts of the first battle in 2021, my darling wife Lorraine told me I had to take my own advice: "Think positive and have faith." That's what I tried to do.

I realize everything I've been through pales in comparison to what these kids go through. I've lived a blessed life. Here I am at 84 years old. This is my fourth quarter. They're just beginning their first quarters. They're a key reason I've been so transparent on social media about my battles. I just want them – and everyone going through cancer – to know they're not alone, because I'm there fighting with them in solidarity.

I'd do anything to fight all the cancer in the world for kids so they don't have to. In that way, I feel like a soldier – a general, even, like my good friend, the late Bob Knight.

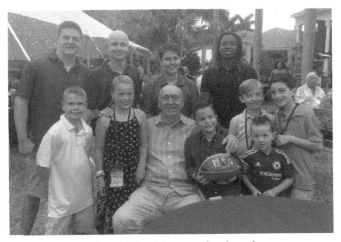

Dick and kids celebrating after the gala.

Know this, cancer: I will fight you until my last breath.

I've learned that to fight the good fight, you need to have a team behind you. Make a militia. Just make sure you're not doing it alone.

I've also learned that while you may need your armor on to fight cancer head on, you can inspire other soldiers (and their families) going through the same fight by taking your armor off and showing them all your emotional scars.

Tony Colton took his armor off to inspire others. So did Jimmy V.

To honor my fourth quarter in life – or overtime, if you will – I'm going to take my own armor off in this book, starting with the next chapter on my latest battle with vocal-cord cancer.

After that lead-off, I'll showcase the strongest kids I know doing the same. First, I'll take you on a journey of where it all began for me: Speaking to a special group of parents who lost their five-year-old girl to cancer. Then I'll visit with a dozen cancer-surviving kids and their families, before spending time with my own. Every chapter will feature a lesson I've learned from these brave kids that applied to my own battles – and hopefully can help others with theirs.

The goal: To show you the unrelenting spirit from these children that inspires me every single day, every single hour, every single minute, every single second.

Until there is no time left on the scoreboard.

To donate to the V Foundation,
Dick Vitale Pediatric Cancer Research Fund,
please scan this code.

Chapter

Two

I Won't be Silenced

with the Dick Vitale Family

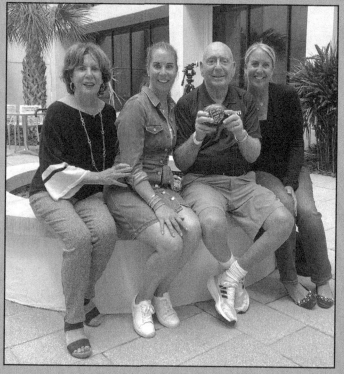

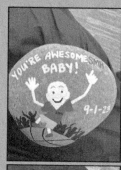

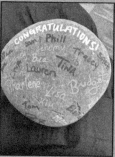

> *"For any cancer treatment, radiation or chemotherapy,
> it's been proven that the more positive your attitude is,
> the better you're able to battle cancer."*
> *- Dr. Matt Biagioli, Dick's radiation oncologist.*

This chapter was written in September of 2023 and kept in its originality.

I feel trapped inside my own body. The monster that is cancer has taken away the most precious gift God gave me.

My voice.

I've made my career, my livelihood, my very name with my voice. And now, as fate would have it, my third bout with cancer has punched me with a knockout blow to the very essence of who I am.

Bitter irony rarely comes so neatly packaged.

That, at least, is the case as I write this. I am hoping against hope that I can soon regain my ability to speak. But, as of now, the voice that has defined me is … gone.

I haven't spoken in over four months. That's because I am resting my vocal cords in the post-treatment phase of laryngeal (vocal-cord) cancer.

I recently concluded 35 grueling radiation treatments spread over six weeks – including a double treatment on Fridays. Nothing about the journey was easy. Doctors told me beforehand I would have swallowing problems to the point where I couldn't eat. (I still did, somehow). My neck had inflammation with a burning sensation like a severe sunburn. Sore throats were an everyday occurrence.

But none of those physical symptoms can compare to the agony I've been in

> *I've made my career, my livelihood, my very name with my voice. And now, as fate would have it, my third bout with cancer has punched me with a knockout blow to the very essence of who I am.*
>
> *- Dick Vitale*

being unable to speak – with my loved ones, my donors who help me raise money for pediatric cancer, my ESPN audience of college hoops fans. Everyone, even with strangers I happen to run into in public places.

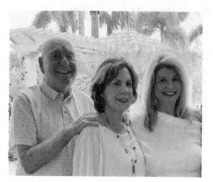

Dick with his sister Terry and Lorraine.

"Talking to people is what brings you the most joy in life," Lorraine tells me. She is my amazing wife of 52 years and has been my rock through all this. There's no way I would be able to handle all the radiation appointments, scans, and bloodwork without her leading the way.

"You've been heartbroken because you're totally healthy in your body besides your voice," she tells me.

"We've been determined to not let cancer take your joy from you."

Lorraine is right. Cancer is the cruelest of diseases because of what it threatens to take from you. I know this now firsthand. It isn't just my voice at stake.

There's no way around this chilling fact: Cancer has the ability to suck the life out of you – physically, mentally and emotionally. Fighting the disease demands the around-the-clock commitment of a full-time job. Treatments can keep it from spreading, but it takes more than that to fend off the horrendous mental anguish that accompanies cancer.

My sister Terry tells me: "If someone were to tell me that my brother was to lose his voice, Richie, I'd tell them it's the equivalent of you losing your life. Growing up into now I can't remember you ever saying you *can't* do something or it's *too difficult*. But this is the toughest battle you've ever had to face because it threatens to take away your purpose."

This is the toughest battle you've ever had to face because it threatens to take away your purpose.

-Terry Vitale, Dick's sister

Do I have my dark moments? You're damn right I do. But through the darkness, I reach back to my late parents, John and Mae, who always told me: *Never Believe in Can't, Richie.*

My beautiful family has been my life support through all of this, led by Lorraine. She will always be my Cinderella story. (I'm the No. 16 seed, of course.) My daughters, Terri and Sherri, have been by my side every step of the way, along with Terri's husband, Chris Sforzo, and Sherri's, Thomas Krug.

And of course, I have my five amazing grandchildren – Sydney, Connor, Jake, Ryan, and Ava – to keep me young with their endless positive energy.

Most notably, I hone in on Jimmy V's words that resound in my heart more than ever and speak to me personally now. They are words that only cancer battlers and survivors – like the brave kids who headline this book – can truly grasp: *"Cancer can take away all my physical abilities. But it cannot touch my mind, it cannot touch my heart, and it cannot touch my soul. Those three things are going to carry on forever."*

Jimmy, my man, cancer has taken away my most cherished physical ability: My voice. But I won't let it reach my mind, my heart, or my soul. I promise you that, my good friend.

Jimmy and I were both coaches. So, in preparing for a daunting opponent, coaches know that strategy is essential. The game plan I've come to use this time has been a credit to lessons I've learned from all the childhood cancer survivors in this book, as well as wisdom I gained from my first two battles with melanoma and lymphoma.

The strategy first emphasizes that you cannot underestimate your opponent. In other words, you gotta allow yourself to briefly feel the heartache and pain that cancer intends to wreak on your body and mind. It would be a

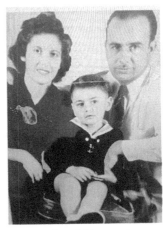

Dick with his parents John and Mae.

mistake to pretend cancer isn't a formidable opponent in this way. Sharing your suffering along the way can also help others not feel so alone.

Allow yourself to feel all that, but only briefly. Then you *must* quickly land your counter punch: Do not let cancer pull you down. Do not let it keep you in a negative mindset. Fight – and fight like hell – to stay positive and muster enough hope.

"You've always taught us, Dad, that life is 1 percent about what's happened to you and 99 percent how you respond to it," my daughter Terri reminds me. "It's about having a lot of little wins add up to become the big win."

It's so true. Taking on cancer is more of a marathon than a sprint. And your mindset at each milepost matters. I keep reminding myself: The comeback is stronger than the setback.

"For any cancer treatment, radiation or chemotherapy, it's been proven that the more positive your attitude is, the better you're able to battle cancer," my radiation oncologist, Dr. Matt Biagioli, says. "If you're anxious and don't have a support system to regulate you, then the cortisol levels can suppress your immune system and your body's ability to eliminate cancer cells goes down."

Trust me on this: You cannot attain positivity without external help. For me, that's been in the form of faith and family. In this latest fight, it's been crucial that I stay active with them. To accomplish this, I'd fit in two naps a day so I would have the energy to go out and be around friends and family amidst my radiation treatments. Routine has also been huge for me – not letting cancer take away my morning breakfasts or my travel plans with family.

"I think you're dealing with cancer like you've dealt with most things in your life: you're facing it head-on," my daughter Sherri says. "You're not letting the diagnosis, treatments or side effects cripple any of us in the family, you're attacking daily life. That's sending a really valuable life lesson to kids and people that life isn't always smooth and it will throw you curveballs, no matter who you are. But it's *how* you respond. You're not acting like everything is all positive. You're facing a painful truth and *then* choosing to be positive."

> *Life isn't always smooth and it will throw you curveballs, no matter who you are. But it's how you respond. You're not acting like everything is all positive. You're facing a painful truth and then choosing to be positive.*
>
> *- Sherri Vitale, Dick's daughter*

I'm done with radiation, but I've needed to harness my positive mindset more than ever lately. Because cancer doesn't stop polluting your thoughts once treatments conclude. No, the disease will attempt to poison your mind during times when hope starts to wane as you don't have answers.

Imagine crossing a finish line for a race and then being told you have to wait for results to determine whether or not all your hard work paid off. That's the scenario I find myself in: Dr. Biagioli told me that since my vocal cords are so sore from all the radiation, we have to wait patiently to see if I'm 100 percent cancer-free.

"You have a very different finish line than most of my patients, Dick," the good doctor tells me. "For you, it isn't just about getting rid of the cancer. It's getting your voice back to normal so that you can do what you love – speak."

The early scopes by Dr. Biagioli have come back positive, but I won't be given a definitive "cancer-free" statement – those golden words cancer patients yearn to hear – until it's certain when I meet with Dr. Steven Zeitels, my otolaryngologist (vocal cord doctor) for the last 15 years. He's the director of Massachusetts General Hospital and renowned for all of his innovative tools and techniques. He's been credited for helping to save the voices of Adele and of Steven Tyler, among others. Heck, I don't even sing.

"We had treated the (pre-cancerous) dysplasia back in 2022 but it was never determined to be cancer," Zeitels says of my case. "Then in July (of 2023) when we examined your vocal cords, I became very worried at what I saw. I eventually saw carcinoma. If you were going to have a shot at keeping your voice, I knew you'd need a combination of microsurgery and radiation."

When you're a cancer patient, the agony of waiting to find out if your chemo or radiation is successful is almost worse than the actual diagnosis or treatment because of how mentally and emotionally exhausting it can be. The waiting game absolutely sucks.

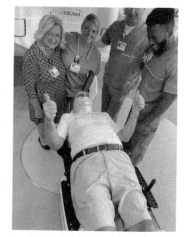

Dick with a radiation mask on.

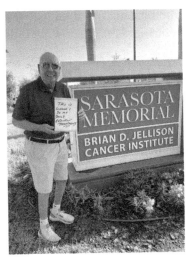

Dick outside the hospital where he fought vocal-cord cancer.

That's why when the cancer clouds surround you, it's vital to have something you love to do, something you're passionate about, as a driving force to get yourself out of the often-suffocating fog.

If I'm blessed to be able to ring the bell of being cancer-free a third time here in the coming weeks, then I'd pivot to work with Dr. Zeitels to try to manage my vocal cords in time so that I can call college basketball games for ESPN sometime in 2024. I'm told I will have a voice when it's all said and done with treatments, but how much I can project – which is crucial for broadcasting – is another waiting game.

"Since I've known you, Dick, you've had this ability to get very upset about your circumstances but then your mind and your passion take over," Zeitels says. "It's like watching a boxer get knocked down in a prize fight and you wonder if he's gonna get up or not. You surprise me, but you always do get up. My prediction is whatever happens (with the exam), you won't be stopped from doing what you set out to do because of the power of your passion."

Now I understand that at 84 years old, clinging to the hope of calling college basketball games once again, it's easy to say, "Gee whiz, why does he need more at that age, why doesn't he retire and enjoy himself?" Well, to those pundits I'd say that I truly enjoy myself sitting courtside. That's my enjoyment. That's not *work*. My father *worked*. What do I do? I sit at a game, in the best seat in the house, get paid, and I watch basketball – talking about a game I love to all my buddies watching on their home screens.

And as of this stage, no doctor has told me to retire. I've asked plenty of experts if it makes sense for me to step down. They tell me that I'm healthy otherwise and my mind is too sharp to step aside from doing something I love to do.

"The depression and anxiety I've seen you experience doesn't seem to be tied to the fear of dying," Dr. Biagioli says. "It's more tied to the fear of not being able to do what you love, what makes you *you*."

When I've been down in the dumps battling cancer, my thoughts drift to the excitement I'd have before calling college hoops games – the goosebumps I'd get when I hear fans chanting, "Dickie V, Dickie V." It's become a part of me for 45 years. That's more than half my life.

When something is taken away that's almost a part of you, it can have a demoralizing effect, let me tell you. So, yeah, fighting to get that part of me back has been at the forefront of my motivation.

When we were little, you used to tell us to never let adversity stop us from chasing our dreams. By fighting to do what you love near the end of your life, you're showing kids to do the same at the beginning of theirs.

- Terri Vitale, Dick's Daughter

"When we were little, you used to tell us to never let adversity stop us from chasing our dreams," my daughter Terri reminds me. "By fighting to do what you love near the end of your life, you're showing kids to do the same at the beginning of theirs."

That's what this is truly all about. Three diagnoses may have thrust me into this position, but my heart's been in this fight far longer. I am in the fight against cancer – all cancers, but childhood cancers most especially. I'm most cut up inside emotionally from being sidelined as a coach to my All-Courageous Team of young cancer survivors and the countless others we can influence. No voice means no working the phones to try to raise money from donors for pediatric cancer. These kids need their advocate, their general, fighting on the front lines.

> *Cancer has silenced my greatest weapon to fight for children by attacking my vocal cords. I feel like Clark Kent without the ability to turn into Superman. My voice is my superpower, baby!*
>
> *- Dick Vitale*

Cancer has silenced my greatest weapon to fight for children by attacking my vocal cords. I feel like Clark Kent without the ability to turn into Superman. My voice is my superpower, baby!

"In a way, your superpower – your voice, and the overuse of it – is what caused the cancer or your Kryptonite," Dr. Biagioli says.

I won't stop wearing my cape if I get it back, though. If anything, I'm just praying I can turn my own fight into a positive for these kids – to show their superpower of courageousness even more.

"I think before you had cancer, you naturally were able to empathize with their parents because you could imagine what it was like for

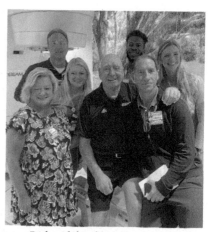

Dick with his doctors and nurses.

them as if it were one of your kids or grandkids," my brother John says. "But since getting cancer yourself, now you can see what the kids are really going through. You understand their world a little better."

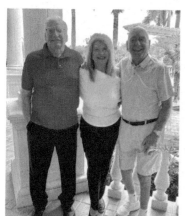

Dick with his brother John and sister Terry.

John's sure right. We're in the same world of aches and pains. Remember, it's not just horrible chemo treatments that these kids face. It's all kinds of aches and pains, endless tests and pokes with needles, countless headaches. And, most of all, the loss of normalcy and fun.

For 15 years prior to my first diagnosis with cancer, in 2021, I had been pleading to raise money for these children. Since my diagnosis, we raised $23.5 million from my two galas. In just two years we raised one third of what we had previously raised in 15. If more dollars for the kids proves to be the silver lining in all of this, then that's a win in my book.

"Your own cancer may limit you physically, but I think it's only intensified your will to fight for these kids," Lorraine says. "In that way, your voice is louder than ever."

My wife is a smart lady.

The reality is I have only lost my voice in the talk-out-loud sense. I still have my voice in the take-on-cancer sense.

This book *is* my voice.

And I see myself as a voice for the voiceless: Kids with cancer who can't speak for themselves.

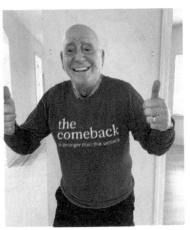

Dick wearing "the comeback is stronger than the setback" shirt.

— Dickie V's Cancer Battle Timeline —

<u>June, 2021:</u> Dick begins several facial procedures to remove melanoma, his first brief bout with cancer.

<u>October, 2021:</u> Doctors determine that Dick has lymphoma, which was misdiagnosed as bile-duct cancer in September, for his second cancer diagnosis. Six months of chemotherapy ensue.

<u>December, 2022:</u> Dick is diagnosed with pre-cancerous dysplasia and ulcerous lesions – a separate diagnosis from the lymphoma – prompting him to go on voice rest – for the first time – for three months.

<u>April, 2022:</u> Dick rings the bell and is declared cancer-free from his lymphoma. That same month, he concludes his voice rest with the dysplasia healed.

<u>July, 2023:</u> Dick is diagnosed with laryngeal (vocal-cord) cancer, his third time battling cancer. Six weeks of radiation treatment ensue.

<u>October, 2023:</u> Dick is determined to be cancer-free after his radiation concluded and his voice healed.

Chapter Three
Unbeatable Positivity
with the Payton Wright Family

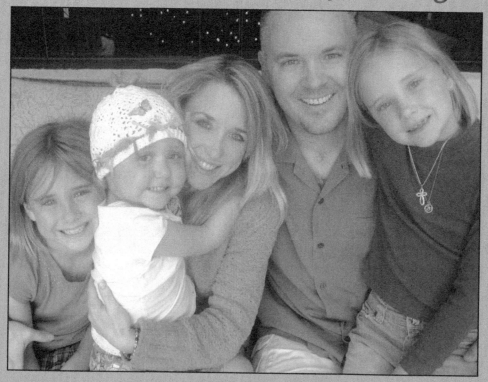

"Payton's message was,
'It's okay. You'll get through it.
It's gonna be a good day, regardless.' "
- Patrick Wright

"Don't worry, Daddy. It's gonna be a good day."

That's what an adorable little girl by the name of Payton Wright told her father, Patrick, when she was wheeled into her first surgery and caught him crying. An MRI had revealed cancerous tumors in Payton's spine and pelvis.

It was a regular occurrence for Payton to inspire others – children and adults alike – during her courageous cancer battle. At the children's hospital, when 10-year-old kids would be consumed by fear before going into daunting chemotherapy or radiation treatments for the first time, she would have the nurses bring her wheelchair up to those kids. She'd give them a pep talk about how it was going to be okay and that they could get through it.

She was just four years old then.

When I talk passionately about fighting against pediatric cancer, you have to know that it all started with Payton. Her inspiration is tattooed on my heart forever.

Patrick and Holly, Payton's parents, live in Lakewood Ranch, Florida. That's where Lorraine and I live, too, so we're practically neighbors. We'd always see Payton at the Broken Egg restaurant, sometimes wearing a little bit of Tinkerbell makeup and lighting up the room with her smile. She loved to watch *Finding Nemo* while eating goldfish crackers and she'd always be a jokester, wearing clown noses around her house. She also loved to be a protector to her older sisters, Savanna and Sydney. She was a special little girl who had a zest for life that was contagious, to say the least.

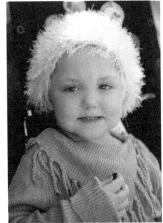

Payton always lit up the room.

I first met Payton in 2006, shortly after she was diagnosed with medulloepithelioma – a rare form of brain cancer that at the time had no treatment protocol and offered very little hope for recovery.

The instant connection began when a family friend showed up at my front door with Payton. They said they read about an event we had at our house raising money for adult cancer with the V Foundation and asked if I could do something to help the family. I offered a personal donation but told them I couldn't do another fundraiser so quickly after the previous one.

The disappointment on her face kept me up all night, tossing and turning, only wishing there was something I could do for this beautiful youngster fighting for her life. I talked all night with Lorraine determined that we must do something to help the Wrights.

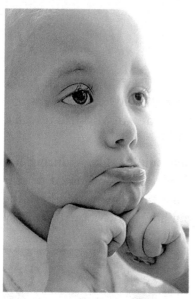

Payton making a face.

The next day, I contacted them and said, "Look, it won't be a big bash but we want to host an event at our house to help raise money for personal expenses." One thing important to realize is that it's tough, if not impossible, for Moms and Dads to focus on a job when your four-year-old daughter is in the battle of her life.

The fundraiser exceeded expectations and raised over $100,000. That was truly the genesis of my annual galas. It all started at my house before we moved the event to the Ritz Carlton to seat over 900 people and have some major celebrity guests over the years: Derek Jeter, Jeff Gordon, John McEnroe, Nick Saban, Dabo Swinney, Pat Summitt, and a laundry list of my iconic men's college basketball coaching friends.

All of it started because of Payton. Her story, like so many others, is equal parts heartbreaking and inspirational.

It's one thing to hear about how glowing this little bald girl was in public when her family would be at restaurants, how brave she was as she'd talk about the rocks in her head that were making her sick (what she called her tumors). But it's another thing to think about how bad a four-year-old girl was hurting as she just begged for the pain to stop. It's these dark moments of suffering that capture why I care so much, and why I wear my heart on my sleeve fighting for these courageous kids.

The day of that first fundraiser at our house came after the Wrights had traveled back from another brutal round of Payton's chemotherapy at Duke's Children's Hospital in Durham, N.C. We tried to make the day extra special for the party. My daughters, Terri and Sherri, decorated the house like you would for a four-year-old's birthday bash.

After about an hour into the party, Payton began screaming that she wanted to go home because she was in so much pain. We didn't know it at the time, but that pain was coming from the tumor compressing her spinal cord. Her cancer had returned and metastasized. The next day, Payton was flown back to Durham and eventually became paralyzed from the waist down.

I've heard that type of screaming before. It was with Jimmy V at a hotel in Bristol, Conn., outside of ESPN studios. Jimmy would compare it to a toothache, except going through his entire system. To know that a little kid was going through the same type of pain ripped my heart in half.

It wasn't the only time I heard Payton's screams, but those first ones remain pierced on my heart because that was the first time I could see her suffering up close.

"I think it was that night," Holly says, "that you really got to meet *cancer*. You really saw the pain part of it that night."

She's right. I didn't just see Payton that night. No, I saw an opponent. A hideous opponent picking on a kid.

I think about Payton's tears from that pain a lot, if I'm being honest. I thought about her grit and tenacity when I was going through my own chemotherapy treatments for lymphoma in 2021 into 2022. When I'd lay in my hospital bed, after my family would leave me, all kinds of thoughts would race through my head. The thoughts can get ugly, let me tell you.

When I was at my worst pain and my body ached all over, I'd refocus my thoughts and think about how courageous Payton was facing terminal cancer. Then I'd start to think of why I need to be strong – to do all I can within my power to lead a fight for kids just like Payton. These kids needed their general in their fight. So I *needed* to get better.

That ability to recalibrate your thinking is not easy. So much of getting through a cancer battle is psychological. It's your mindset. I know that now firsthand as I've created my own motto: Think positive and have faith.

It's gonna be a good day."
- Payton Wright

The Wrights know a thing or two about mindset. They dealt with blow after blow, almost losing Payton several times. It was August of 2006 when she became paralyzed from the waist down. Cancer later spread all over to the point where Payton lost most of her vision.

One thing that always floored me was how the Wrights would redirect their focus after devastating setbacks, almost like a GPS that lost its original tracking. They'd dig down deep and find a perspective that no one else could see.

I will never forget the phone call I got from Patrick when my entire family was at the Atlantis resort in the Bahamas for a vacation. Talk about polar opposite of realities. I was sitting poolside with Lorraine observing our five grandkids having a blast going down water slides. When Patrick called, he was so excited. Payton was at Duke Children's Hospital at the time and both he and Holly were hoping for a miracle. He called to tell me that after undergoing all the radiation a human body can handle, doctors agreed to get Payton into a wheelchair so Patrick and Holly could take her for breakfast outside. She had a few bites before getting sick, but Patrick was ecstatic just to take her outside.

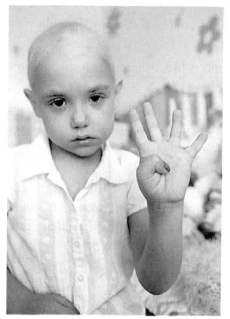

Payton holding up the number four.

That perspective was a splash of cold water in my face. The contrast was striking. Are you kidding me? That's a father not taking anything for granted right there.

I was crying like a baby when I got off the phone and said to Lorraine, "Life can be so unfair." We were out having a fabulous time with our family on vacation while Patrick was thrilled simply because he could go to breakfast outside with his little girl.

It changes your life when your child has cancer. The way you think, the way you act, everything. But that mindset shift takes willpower, baby. The most serious kind.

"The little things start to matter more," Patrick says. "You don't take days for granted anymore. What Payton taught us and can teach others was that you could be going through something, it doesn't have to be cancer. It could be someone you love dying, grieving in a divorce, fighting through an addiction. Payton's message was, 'It's okay. You'll get through it. It's gonna be a good day, regardless.' "

Patrick and Holly say they didn't speak for two weeks after Payton's initial diagnosis. Then they decided how to take on their daughter's cancer as a true team. That is easier said than done. These are the types of tragedies that can throttle a marriage and family dynamic. Not with the Wrights, though.

Lorraine and I sat in awe at their teamwork. Holly would focus on the attunement and caretaking. Patrick would focus on navigating what the doctors were saying. Then he would tell Holly any bad news when the time was right, so as to not quell the positive vibes around Payton.

That unyielding positivity Holly showed trickled down into how Payton saw the world – and the people in it.

"We weren't going to let her feel it," Holly says. "She just loved life. She had this mindset of, 'Yeah, this sucks right now.' But then she could name off five other things she was grateful for. And she'd be hooked up to all these cords in chemo but always wanted to talk to others and help them. I really wish I could bottle her up to show everyone. I don't think I have the words to describe her."

I'd hear story after story from the Wrights about how Payton would ooze out strength and happiness in spite of the adversity she faced. One story I love is about how Payton would be so loveable to the medical staff during radiation, listening to rock 'n' roll music (instead of your standard Disney stuff) and bravely go through the treatments.

Like a rock star, baby. I love it.

"Kids would wear a type of mask for radiation," Holly says. "So we'd practice (the radiation process) with her beforehand by putting a wash cloth on her face, she'd take deep breaths and focus on the song. The doctors couldn't believe she wasn't sedated."

She wore a facemask for radiation, just like she put on a brave face for visitors. Yet it's the times when I saw Payton without her mask that haunt me and drive me. Those times when she couldn't help but cry out.

At four and five years old, Payton didn't know psychologically how bad her diagnosis was, but there would be times where she'd be feeling pain – unbearable pain I'd see at our house with my own eyes – and be brought to tears. Lorraine and I would see her at her bravest moments.

That's why anytime I saw her, I would often put on a brave mask myself and be as cordial as you could with a four or five-year-old. Later I would break down in tears as I thought about all Payton was going through, all Holly and Patrick and Savanna and Sydney were going through.

Payton saw things differently. She wasn't going to have bad days. Again, she had a powerful perspective.

"Her spirit was definitely one of an old soul," Holly says. "In treatment, she'd be talking to the nurses and knew all this medical terminology. They walked out and thought they were talking to a 30-year-old. She had this type of resolve."

I get emotional when I hear Holly pay me the grandest of compliments. "Payton had this Dickie V feistiness about her. She was bold, a little sassy, and would talk to anyone. Her presence was known when she came into the room."

Patrick recalls the close bond I had with Payton: "We'd be at a restaurant for a dinner and you would have a microphone, Dick. You'd be talking about her like she was a celebrity. She'd say, 'Is that Mr. V talking about me again?' and smile."

That gives me chills just remembering it all.

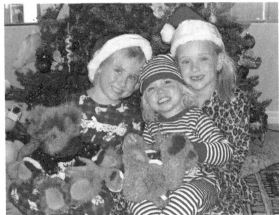

Payton with her sisters.

"Now she's working within you, fighting through you, Dick," Holly tells me.

Wow. Talk about an honor. Especially coming from Payton, one of my biggest heroes in life. Because that's what she is to me: A true hero.

Payton's death ignited something in my heart that won't ever go away now. She played a keen role in me developing an absolute obsession to get grants to create new medications and treatments for children.

- Dick Vitale

I put her fighting spirit right in line with some of my adult heroes. What Payton did in her cancer fight is what Jimmy V did in his, without even knowing she was taking my man's advice. For Jimmy, not giving up was about getting up on that stage at the ESPYs. For Payton, it was graduating her preschool class in May of 2007.

She never gave up.

All up until May 29, 2007, when the cancer had spread and took Payton from us. She was just five years old.

Patrick and Holly tell me that people at the church funeral service complained they couldn't hear because I was weeping so loudly. I couldn't help it. Listening to Holly speak up there about her little angel showing pictures of Payton when she was healthy at the beach, and playing with her older sisters, was so heartbreaking.

After the service, Lorraine and I ran to find Holly and Patrick after the funeral procession in the crowd of people. I said to them, "I will not let her pass without Payton helping other kids." I told them then I would raise over $1 million for a research grant in her name. When Lorraine and I got into our car, she said to me: "Do you realize what you just committed to do?" I said to her, "Lorraine, we will get it done."

Payton's death ignited something in my heart that won't ever go away now. She played a keen role in me developing an absolute obsession to get grants to create new medications and treatments for children.

Payton's battle reminds me of what my late colleague Stuart Scott said during his 2014 ESPYs speech. He said, "When you die, it does not mean that you lose to cancer. You beat cancer by how you live, why you live, and in the manner in which you live. So, live, fight like hell. And when you get too tired to fight, then lay down and rest and let somebody else fight for you."

Payton did just that with her fight. And not only did she beat cancer by that definition, but now she's beating it via her legacy that continues to save other kids' lives. She's letting us fight for her now.

Here's an example of how Payton's legacy has lived on in a very practical way since her passing. One of my All-Courageous team members, Kyle Peters, had a similar type of brain cancer to Payton's. The money raised through Payton's research grant helped doctors manage Kyle's care. Today he is the coordinator of Florida Operations for the Pittsburgh Pirates.

"That makes me feel so proud of my precious daughter, but hearing that is like an emotional roller coaster," Holly says. "I remember crying that, finally, we are helping children with cancer. Finally, we are putting pediatric cancer on the map. I also had tears of, 'Why couldn't this be done years ago, so that my child had more of a chance to survive?' "

There's a reason every dollar I raise, including every profit from this book, goes to pediatric cancer research. Because these kids need it.

After my gala in 2007, Bob Knight's wife, Karen, came up to Holly and told her that her brother had similarly died of brain cancer, in 1956. She said everything her brother went through was the same as Payton's.

"When Payton was diagnosed, I didn't think my child was going to die," Holly says. "I didn't know that the same procedures they were using in 1956 they were using on my kid in 2006. I was sick when I heard that. Appalled they haven't come up with anything new."

Now they have. Thanks to Payton.

One takeaway I hope to convey is that Payton was a leader in this world, and she inspires me to be a leader in her name.

"These other kids need a leader now," Holly says. "They need a coach, a role model. It doesn't surprise me that you're fighting in this pediatric arena. Because your makeup has always been doing everything you can for kids – of all ages."

> *I didn't know that the same procedures they were using in 1956 were being used on my kid in 2006. I was sick when I heard that. Appalled they haven't come up with anything new.*
>
> *- Holly Wright*

All the grieving parents – all the Patrick and Holly Wrights of the world – need a leader, too. I want to make sure that all of the Moms and Dads don't have their children forgotten. This fight is to honor them just as much as future cancer battlers.

"We know it's okay to be broken," Patrick says of his ongoing grief. "Because we're still broken. We're never going to get over Payton's loss. Grief doesn't stop. We're often wondering what Payton would look like today, in her 20s. What college would she be going to, what sports would she have played."

But Patrick says one key part of managing grief is you don't give up in that area, either. You don't force yourself to forget.

"In that way, we're listening to Payton now in our own fight," Patrick says. "We have pictures all over the place in our home and always toast to her, tell funny stories and cry and reminisce. It keeps her spirit alive with us. Payton's older sisters wanted to have a seat with Payton's picture in it at the family table for their weddings. Every family gathering, you have that feeling in the back of your mind that one's not there."

Holly agrees fighting through grief isn't easy. But she's got her little angel guiding her – and Patrick and Savanna and Sydney – through that.

"Payton wasn't ever giving up," she says. "When she was first diagnosed, she was given five weeks. She made it a whole year. That right there proves her will. The child couldn't slow down, even with the chemo, even with being paralyzed. She fought until the very end."

Yes, Payton is gone, but her legacy lives on. Make no mistake.

Patrick and Holly often tell me this fight against pediatric cancer is draining for me. Working on adult cures instead would've been a lot easier, they say. "You're constantly loving on sick kids," Patrick says.

They're right, baby. I won't stop fighting. That's my way of honoring Payton, until cancer is cured for all kids just like her. And Lorraine is right there with me.

We won't give up.

Because Payton never did.

Patrick and Holly Wright raise money to support cancer-stricken families through The Payton Wright Foundation, assisting families just like them when work is the last thing to think about during a child's cancer battle. Their website is paytonwright.org

To donate to the V Foundation,
Dick Vitale Pediatric Cancer Research Fund,
please scan this code.

Chapter Four

Defeating Relapse

with the Weston Hermann Family

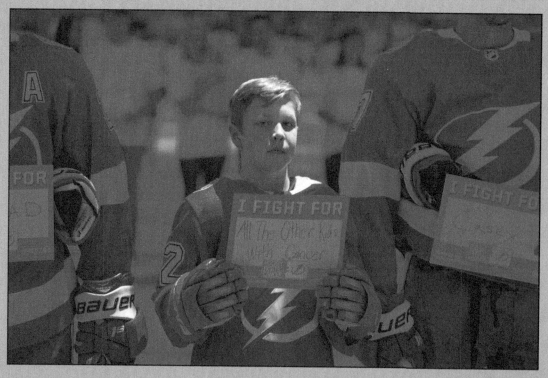

In pro hockey, we have some of the toughest customers in all of sports and the Stanley Cup is arguably the hardest to win. That mental toughness pales in comparison to Weston battling cancer four separate times. Or any kid battling cancer. Wins and losses are not life and death."
- Tampa Bay Lightning Coach Jon Cooper

Every Wednesday, for more than a year, Weston Hermann treated his chemotherapy treatments as if they were hockey games.

"The way I looked at it," he tells me, "there was a winner and a loser. I wasn't about to lose any of those weeks."

That was the mindset of this iron-willed boy, then 13, for 55 consecutive weeks of dreaded Wednesday chemotherapy sessions, always at 1 p.m. sharp.

Weston approached his physical battle with a unique mental fervor – treating his brain cancer as a beatable opponent, one that he had every intention of dominating.

Today, at 17, he is one of the best hockey players of his age in Florida. That is partly because he never stopped playing while undergoing chemo. In fact, he would regularly go directly from chemo to practice. Of course he did. The ice rink was his sanctuary, a place where he didn't have to think about the rigors of cancer. Even if sometimes it meant puking in the parking lot before getting out on the ice.

He played in a hockey game right after his first chemo session – and recorded three goals and two assists. My man Weston is downright inspiring, baby, playing through that pain in a weakened state. That is Michael Jordan Flu Game-level toughness right there.

"I really looked at my entire cancer battle as a hockey game," he says. "For me, it all kind of ran on the same system because at the end of the day, you just have to focus on winning. You have to take things play by play, period by period."

Or, in his case, relapse by relapse.

The course of Weston's battle with cancer came in four stages. Think of it as the three periods of a hockey game, plus overtime.

He was first diagnosed in January 2014, when he was 7. Weston began treatment at Boston Children's Hospital – where his brother, Grayson, was being treated for his heart. In the same weekend that Grayson went in for cardiac surgery, Weston went in for brain surgery. Grayson's procedure was a success, while doctors thought they had gotten rid of Weston's tumor completely.

Turned out it was only the first period for Weston.

FACT:
75 percent of childhood cancer survivors have at least one chronic health condition and 40 percent have life-threatening conditions by 30 years of age.
- Journal of the American College of Cardiology

Cancer recurred in April of 2016, when he was 9, prompting 14 months of chemotherapy. (Those, by the way, were his first set of chemo sessions.) When he completed those, in 2017, he rang the bell. Everyone hoped that meant he was done with cancer, but that bell was really just a horn to signal the end of the second period.

"As soon as you have a doctor say to you, 'Can we step outside for a minute?' – you know it's something bad," says Weston's father, Jared Hermann. "It's this nightmare that keeps happening on replay."

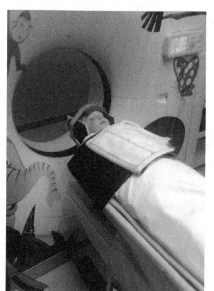

In November of 2017, Weston had his second brain surgery. Both of those surgeries "were difficult decisions because his tumor was located on the left side of his motor strip," Jared says. "Doctors told us that for the first surgery, there was a 50 percent probability of paralysis on the left side. That significantly increased to 70 to 75 percent probability in the next surgery."

That one was completed at Children's Hospital of Philadelphia. Doctors again hoped this would wipe out Weston's cancer for good. It seemed like the end of the third period.

If only.

Weston's overtime, his fourth run-in with brain cancer, came in May 2020 – two months after the national lockdown from the pandemic.

Weston in treatment.

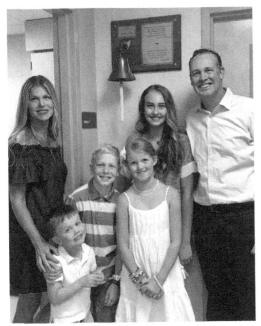

Weston rings the bell with the support of his family.

That's when those 55 rounds of chemo began. I know those returned diagnoses took a toll on Jared, stepmother Aimée, Weston's mother, Marcie, and all his siblings – Makenna, Charlée (14) and Grayson (12).

Weston rang his (hopefully final) bell again in July of 2021 – and has been cancer-free ever since.

"Each battle, each period, you get tougher mentally," Weston says. "Once you know you can do it once, then you know you can do it again. Once you get through it twice, you feel confident from that. Then when it happens again, you've gotten through it three times. I knew I would beat it. When you face cancer, you have to have a good mentality. If you're not in the right state of mind, it can get the upper hand."

Weston used hockey metaphors throughout his fight. Naturally, I use basketball metaphors for mine. When I battled lymphoma in 2021-22, I treated remission as my Final Four and getting my voice back from dysplasia that year as my national championship.

That ability Weston has reconfiguring his mental battle – not playing the "why me" card after a relapse – is beyond impressive. I, too, thought I was out of the woods after ringing the bell in the spring of 2022. Then, for cancer to come back in a different way a year later, it was just devastating. I have deepened empathy for Jared's notion of a nightmare on repeat.

In my 35 radiation treatments over six weeks in 2023, I didn't allow myself to meander in frustrated emotions from getting cancer a third time, as badly as I wanted to. Because my man Weston didn't take the complain train with his relapses. I couldn't help but think of his determination. Talk about inspiring, baby.

Weston's hockey-minded resolve offered me a playbook. It's almost like a fellow coach sharing game tape of an opponent. He tells me it's finding the little things to focus on, counting the little "wins," so to speak, that can help you get through it all – the Wednesdays at 1 p.m., in his case.

To combat the taste of the chemo, Weston would eat lemons or Warheads Sour Candy. It's these small, creative tactics that helped him know the chemo wasn't going to mess with his taste – or his psyche.

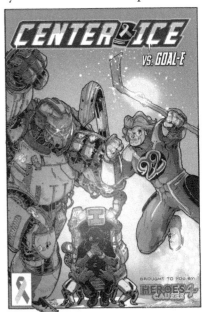

Weston's comic book.

On the heels of being cancer-free, Weston created a comic book called *Center Ice*. The hero wears a No. 22 hockey sweater – Weston's number, of course. The villain is Mr. I, as in the MRIs that were once Weston's nemesis. Now the comic book can be found in many hospitals around the country.

"My battle with cancer can help me mentally with anything I face in life," Weston says. "It's an experience not a lot of other people have and something I can use as motivation. It makes some of these other life challenges feel easier."

Weston's approach to life wasn't always what it is today. It took fine-tuning over time. You gotta remember: Getting cancer treatments – the adult kinds – when you're a kid is traumatic, to say the least.

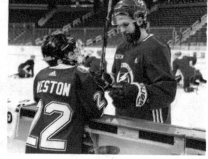

"It was tough at first," Jared recalls. "We didn't even use the C-word with him that first time around. The hardest part as a father is you feel like you lose your ability to protect your child. The first round of chemo was traumatic for him and changed his personality during treatments at the hospital.

"There was one point where I was chasing him around the hospital halls, and he'd be restraining from doctors or nurses putting chemo in

Weston practicing with the Lightning.

his port. …He got used to getting knocked down and having to get back up at a young age and that's carried over into today."

Sometimes, it's in the how we get back up. I think one thing Weston and I have in common is how we use the sport we love – youth hockey for him, college basketball for me – as motivators in our cancer battles.

"We found it more mentally advantageous for him to play hockey than the worries of him physically falling down and hurting his head, so he was limited, but being on the ice and a part of a team was what we decided to have him do," Jared says.

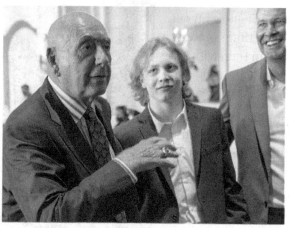

Weston with Dick at his gala.

The sport turned out to be the best medicine of all.

"If I didn't have hockey or it was taken away from me, I wouldn't be able to have the mindset I've had," Weston says. "Having hockey gave me something to look forward to, somewhere to escape to – but also something to want to get better for. Having something to push for and look to the future for can completely change everything in how you face cancer."

He's so right about this. Heck, why do you think I'm still trying to call games at 84? I'm trying to be the first

100-year-old broadcaster, baby! The reality is I still get chills when I walk into stadiums. So, you see, the first thing I asked Dr. Zeitels when he told me I'd be trapped without my voice again was: Will I be able to call games for ESPN for my 45th season? I was already thinking ahead.

But here I am in the twilight of a blessed career, a blessed life. Weston's got his whole future in front of him. And, oh my, how bright it is. He's been on the ice since he was 6 and has dreamed of playing in the NHL ever since – before cancer ever hit him.

"I thought at some point, he'd get burnt out on the sport," Jared says. "But his passion seems to grow every single day."

That childhood dream isn't out of reach. First, Weston says he's got to get to the Division I college level; that's his goal for the immediate future. At 17, he stars for the Florida Alliance, a Class AAA program,

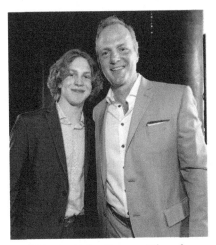

Weston with Jon Cooper at the gala.

and as a freshman he led the Manatee Admirals in goals in the Lightning High School Hockey League.

He's gotten a snapshot of what it would be like to play in the NHL, thanks to an awesome assist from my good friend Jon Cooper, the head coach of the Tampa Bay Lightning. Coop has invited Weston out to practice, Lightning players have taken him on a team fishing trip, and he's dropped the first puck at Lightning games before thousands of fans.

"He was a little guy when I first met him, now he's my height," says Cooper, who guided the Lightning to back-to-back Stanley Cups in 2020 and 2021. The two have gotten close over the years, as Coop is often in lockstep with me fighting cancer in the Tampa community.

"Like you, Dick, I'm left inspired by someone like Weston. Put it this way: In pro hockey, we have some of the toughest customers in all of sports and the Stanley Cup is arguably the hardest to win. That mental toughness required to win pales in comparison to Weston battling cancer four separate times. Or any kid battling cancer. Wins and losses are not life and death."

Weston has been invited to team camps for the United States Hockey League (USHL), North America Hockey League (NAHL), the top amateur levels before the NHL. For him, getting a chance to flourish on the ice is the ultimate win. I love his incredible desire to not let this dreaded disease ever stop him from chasing his dreams.

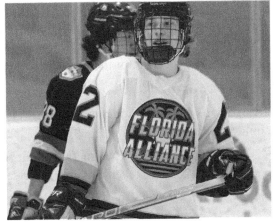

Weston playing for the Florida Alliance.

"The biggest area where he has a leg up, whether it's in hockey or just in life, is his high pain tolerance," Jared says, "The daily obstacles and adversities don't affect him the same way. Because he's basically conquered one of the most challenging (obstacles) anyone would have to face not once, but four times.

"I don't know any other kid who has mental strength from keeping a positive attitude when facing uphill battle after uphill battle."

Jimmy V used to tell me of his own mindset battling cancer: "Put it on the backburner." That's not easy to do when this awful disease feels like it's front row center in your thoughts.

But Weston is a master of the counterattack when adversity hits. He tore two ligaments in his ankle and the doctor said it was a six-month recovery. "He looked at me," Jared says, "and goes, 'He doesn't know me. I'll be back in three months.' "

He was back in 2½ months.

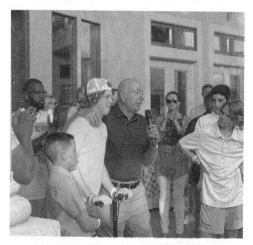

Weston with Dick at the gala picnic.

I first met Jared and Aimée at a restaurant when they approached Lorraine and me to express his appreciation for the dollars we've been raising for pediatric cancer. They sat at our table with us and showed me a video of Weston playing hockey. I was blown away. I feel sick to know the only way to help save their kids is putting chemo toxins in their bodies. Better research on children's cancer will mean they don't have to be treated with outdated regimens intended for adults.

"These drugs are decades and decades old," Jared says. "I had a hard time accepting this stuff being that outdated."

One stat that crushes me: 75 percent of childhood cancer survivors have at least one chronic health condition and 40 percent have life-threatening conditions by 30 years of age. So even in a case like Weston's where he's got his whole future ahead of him, there's concern for the long-term after-effects of what he was forced to do to stay alive.

That needs to change.

Weston's parents tell me how they worry whenever Weston gets a nosebleed, a headache, anything that could signal a relapse.

But that's where he's learning from their son that you don't need to fear cancer when you've beaten it the way he has. It's hard to even consider it a rivalry when you're 4-0 against your opponent.

"Now," Weston tells me, "we gotta beat it for everyone else."

Weston's comic book, Center Ice, can be purchased at Heroesforcauses.com, with the proceeds going to cancer research.

**To donate to the V Foundation,
Dick Vitale Pediatric Cancer Research Fund,
please scan this code.**

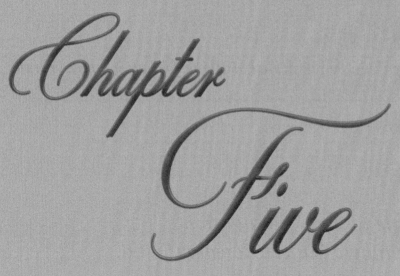

Chapter
Five
You're Not Alone

with the Sadie Keller Family

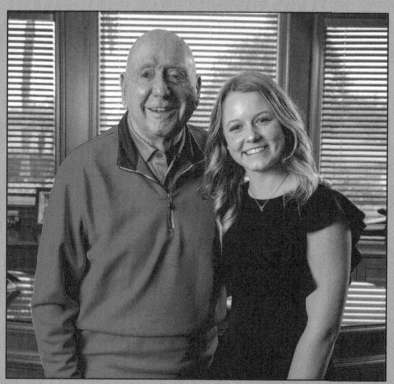

"Kids are the future. Without us, there is no future."
- Sadie Keller

*I*t's not what matters on the outside, it's what matters on the inside.

That is the message of 8-year-old Sadie Keller in one of her first YouTube videos for her series, "What it's like to have cancer as a child."

Sadie was bravely explaining what it was like to lose her hair and go bald during her chemotherapy treatment – emphasizing that one's inner beauty trumps any outer feelings of insecurity.

Let me tell you, my friends, Sadie encapsulated inner beauty in her bout with cancer.

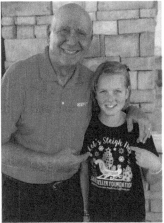

Sadie with Dick at his home.

She was prone to feel anxiety from all of the daunting tests and procedures after she was diagnosed with Acute Lymphoblastic Leukemia at 7. Then she wanted to quell any of those fears for other kids (and their parents) who may have been going through the same emotional roller coaster of tubes and needles. So, quite naturally, she grabbed an iPad and started recording video tutorials in her mother's closet.

"Some people when they get cancer, they get really nervous," she says in her first recording. "I'm gonna try to make it sound easier than what it sounds like to you."

Her videos quickly went viral and were used by ESPN during Jimmy V Week.

That was just the beginning.

Fast forward three years later, on the heels of remission from her three-year battle with cancer, and Sadie had transitioned from her mother's closet to speaking on Capitol Hill. She was lobbying Congress to start investing more in government funding for pediatric cancer research.

"Seven children die each day from childhood cancer," she testified that day. "We must do better. We need more money for research so we can find cures."

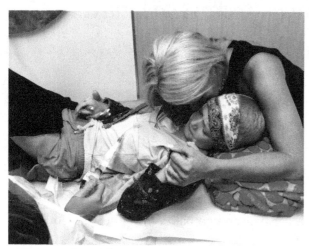

Sadie with her mom during her cancer fight.

Amen, Sadie.

Her cancer story illustrates why research *has* to be better and more catered to children. At the beginning of her treatment, an E.coli infection spread from her shoulder to her chemotherapy port. That meant replacing her port with a painful long-term IV line meant only for adults. A few months in, she started developing stroke-like symptoms. Methotrexate, the medicine being put into her spine – she had 19 spinal taps – to help prevent cancer from spreading had leaked into her brain. That prompted the cells to swell.

"You have the neurologists telling us it's not in our best interest to keep going but then the oncologists telling us we have to keep going because the cancer's going to come back," recalls her father, Shawn.

"It was this rare side effect that was so scary," says Sadie's mother, Sarah. "She was slurring her speech and couldn't say words properly. We had to rally together as a family and make a decision that our No. 1 goal was getting the cancer out first."

These complications don't have to happen if only the procedures are better researched and vetted specifically for children.

"I have the scars on my body to help me remember all the hard times I went through," Sadie tells me.

Sadie has gained wisdom now as a 16-year-old. When you go through weekly chemotherapy treatments for 2 ½ years straight, it undoubtedly grows you up beyond your years.

At 11, Sadie was speaking on television with grit and determination of a woman three times her age. She appeared on CNN's *The Situation Room with Wolf Blitzer*, *NBC Nightly News with Lester Holt* and Fox News's *America's Newsroom*, practically everywhere. She then co-wrote a book with Texas politician Michael McCaul about those who helped her on her fight with cancer. It is called *Better Angels*, and I was honored to be mentioned as one of hers.

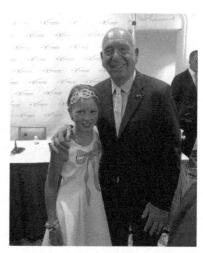

Young Sadie and Dick at one of the many galas she has attended.

The irony is that she's been an angel to Lorraine and me. I knew after seeing her segment on ESPN she was exactly what we were looking for to add a dedicated member to our All-Courageous Team of young cancer survivors. She's been to six of my galas with her family and whenever you meet her, her smile and sincere desire to help others is captivating.

Sadie's the definition of a star and we were so lucky that through our gala she developed a relationship with Mark and Cindy Pentecost, the founders of IT WORKS! They have hearts of gold in the multiple millions of dollars they've donated at the galas. There's no doubt in my mind their friendship with Sadie has played a vital role in raising life-saving dollars.

When I talk to Sadie, she refers to me as a "coach in a fire." Takes one to know one.

"Positivity is what can help you get through cancer, just knowing you can find the good in every situation – no matter how hard," Sadie says.

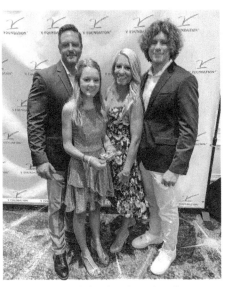

Sadie with her family at the gala.

Shawn and Sarah say the biggest gift, if there is one, from what their family went through, is that they learned to take life's trials day-by-day, hour-by-hour and sometimes minute-by-minute. That's morphed into regular family dinners, memorable trips and a whole lot of "living for today," dating back to Sadie's brother Grant making her laugh when she was feeling ready to cry back during her battle. Nowadays, Sadie's playing tennis cancer-free in front of everyone.

The cancer that got in Sadie's blood at seven years old also seemed to help inject her with the grace to care for others. That's an instinct that may start with a small gesture but carry with it a contagious energy that uplifts people's spirits.

She liked to bake treats for nurses and medical staff, who often don't get enough praise for all that they do. For her

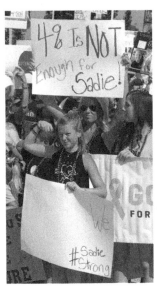

Sadie with her sign at a rally.

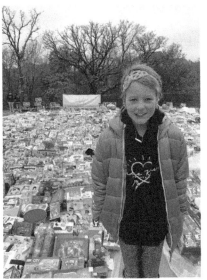

Sadie posing with hundreds of gifts for her foundation.

foundation, she created "Milestone Gifts." These are special somethings set aside to celebrate children having their last chemo or radiation treatments.

The first year she was battling cancer, Sadie got worried about all the other sick kids in Children's Medical Center in Dallas during the holidays. So she created her own fundraiser toy drive that collected thousands of toys for sick children called "Sadie's Sleigh." Through her foundation, since she began in 2015, she's now collected over 100,000 toys for children during Christmas and spread them out over three hospitals in the Dallas-Forth Worth area.

> *It's not what matters on the outside, it's what matters on the inside."*
>
> *- Sadie Keller*

Most importantly, Sadie does all this with a smile as she brings smiles to other youngsters who are in a battle with a disease that she knows too well.

"Christmas is such a happy day and when you're in the hospital, you're not," she says. "I wanted to help as much as I could and make those kids not feel alone."

There it is right there.

It's a point that doesn't get illuminated enough: Cancer can be isolating. It's often the case even if you have a support system of family and friends. The reality is they're not going through what you're going through. It's an inner battle only cancer patients can truly understand.

That's exactly why I did my best to channel Sadie during my own battles with cancer, sharing what I was going through to my nearly 950,000 Twitter (now X) followers.

One of my tweets in March of 2022 said: "This is for those that are in my club of CANCER PATIENTS fighting the journey to beat the disease. Yes, the scans, bloodwork, blood counts, chemo treatments, NEUPOGEN shots that cause intense pain wear on us but remember as my buddy Jimmy V said, 'Don't Give Up…Don't Ever Give Up.'® "

My family gave me a hard time because of how frequently I'd post anything and everything during my cancer battles, but they ultimately knew it was for a greater good. Who needs privacy when you can inspire, baby?

My daughter Terri gets it: "At first it was like, 'Whoa he's really sharing this.' You do that to inspire people who are going through what you're going through. I would argue cancer makes your spirit even stronger."

Sadie knew all about that type of inspiration and spirit.

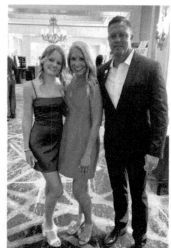

Sadie and her parents at the gala.

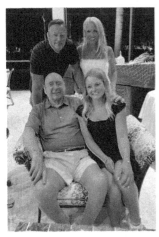

Sadie and her parents with Dick at his home.

When people like Sadie share their feelings publicly, others can understand on a deeper level what it is that a child and family must go through.

Much like Sadie, I felt that by being transparent about my battles versus vocal-cord cancer, lymphoma and melanoma, other cancer-stricken families would not feel so alone. That's why I had no filter: I wanted the truth out there. I tweeted pictures with stories about the various scans, bloodwork and chemotherapy that were a part of my daily routine.

I also wanted to share so that people in the public can understand how the battle entails a full commitment by so many people in your circle. For me, I was able to show how Lorraine is my rock, how blessed I was to have her by my side and how my daughters, Terri and Sherri, and their families, played a pivotal role.

I surely developed a better sense of what these young children like Sadie faced on a regular basis. I figured if I could be vulnerable in my suffering the way that Sadie was, at age eight, people could also grasp this fact: It's one thing for an 84-year-old man to be going through this. It's a whole other battle for children.

"I didn't even know what cancer was," Sadie says. "When you're a child, you're supposed to just play and not know about all these things that grownups know."

Sadie has the physical scars from all the treatment – and the emotional scars, too. Her social life got flipped upside down. She missed most of second grade and virtually all of third grade being homeschooled while going through chemotherapy.

"I missed so much school," she says, "and then when I did get back, everyone was different. I *was* different. Even now, a lot of my friends can't relate to me when I tell them I had childhood cancer. That's tough sometimes when people don't know what to say."

One of the most challenging parts for Sadie was locking onto that message about inner beauty she shared with her followers. "I've watched the videos since and it's hard to watch because I was just a normal little girl (at 8) and you could see I *looked* like I had cancer.

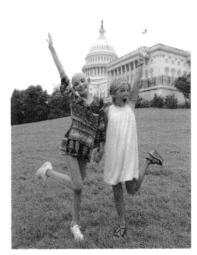

"I lost my hair 7-8 times and that's just so hard as a little girl who wants to have long hair and feel like a girl, feel like everyone else," she says.

In one of her early videos, Sadie adorably tells her viewers: "If someone just brags about being so pretty, they need to be nicer on the inside than on the outside."

Lily and Sadie at the United States Capitol.

It was Sadie's best friend, Lily, who helped her find her inner beauty.

"I first met Lily when I was eight years old and didn't have any hair," Sadie says. "She was done with treatment and a survivor. She told me, 'You just need to keep your confidence up' and told me about her hard times. She became like a mentor. It was so nice to have someone to relate to. We'd FaceTime and text all the time and later lobbied together in Washington."

Lily's cancer unfortunately returned. It's that nightmare so many survivors fear and live with daily even after years in remission.

"When Lily relapsed with her cancer, then I became her mentor and was there for her," Sadie says. "We kind of switched places when I was finishing my battle and she was restarting."

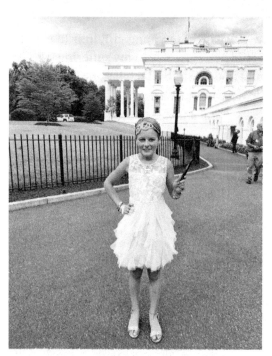

Sadie at The White House with the pen President Trump used to sign the STAR Act.

Sadie gets choked up telling me about Lily's death in 2019: "When she passed away, it was really hard for me. But now I remember all she taught me and how much of a light she was in my life and other people's lives. Now I do what I do because I want to fight for my best friend."

Lily's loss – and what it means to Sadie – is why I feel in lockstep with her goal.

"I've lost so many friends to childhood cancer," she tells me. "We're not only fighting for kids like me, but for friends who passed away. They were too young to pass from something that could've been preventable. I'll remember their stories and never forget them."

I know I have my lane in helping kids like Sadie. I've been blessed through my identity covering college basketball to have a broad reach to help spread awareness. But at the end of the day, what Sadie's doing as a spokeswoman for children fighting cancer everywhere is she's putting a face to the 8 percent. That ugly stat I cannot stand where kids get that mere percentage of funding compared to adult research. She's lobbying several times a year for numerous Childhood Cancer Acts. She already lobbied for the passage of the Creating Hope Act, RACE for Children Act, Global Hope Act, Give Kids A Chance Act, and the STAR Act, the last of which she was invited to the Oval Office for in 2018 when President Donald Trump signed it into law. He handed her the pen after signing – no big deal.

Thanks to the tireless efforts of Sadie and other advocates, we've seen 4 percent of the National Cancer Institute budget vault up to 8 percent. And we still need more.

When I ask her what her message is when she's speaking to Congress, she says it's pretty simple.

"Kids are the future," she says. "Without us, there is no future."

Sadie gives back to families in need through the Sadie Keller Foundation, raising funds for her Milestone gifts or toys in Sadie's Sleigh.
To donate, visit sadiekellerfoundation.org

To donate to the V Foundation, Dick Vitale Pediatric Cancer Research Fund, please scan this code.

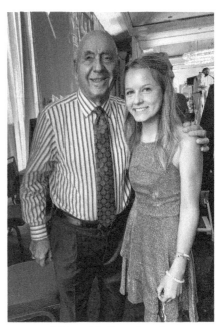

Dick and Sadie at the gala.

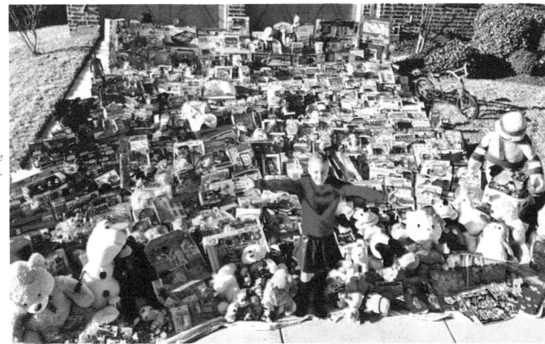

Sadie with the Sadie's Sleigh toys.

Chapter

Six

Suffering for a Purpose

with the Cole Eicher Family

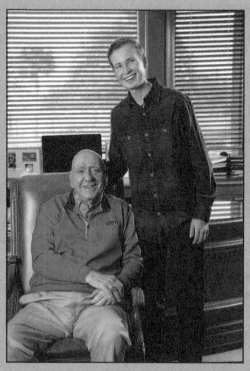

"I'm not afraid to speak to adults about hard topics. God's been training me for this. I'm gonna be their voice."
- Cole Eicher

Cole Eicher tells me the negative thoughts kept on coming, one after the other.

The worst of them, he remembers, came on Good Friday the year he was diagnosed with brain cancer.

Radiation had deteriorated his body's energy. He was vomiting all day and told he'd need a feeding tube to get some food down. Perhaps worse than all the physical symptoms were the emotional ones, with so-called friends overwhelmed and unwilling to support him or stick around.

"Cancer just devastates everything in your life, it puts a pause on everything," says Cole, who was 12 years old when he began a rigorous year-long treatment to address the golf ball-sized medulloblastoma tumor in the back of his brain. He endured 30 radiation treatments, four months of intensive chemotherapy, and brain surgery. That led to an uphill road getting his motor skills and walking ability back to normal.

Cole tells me of his breaking point: "I started asking, 'Why is God doing this to me? This could've happened to anyone else, why me?' I was angry and hurting in every way. In the Bible, it says that God's plan is perfect and to put all of your trust in Him. I realized cancer was affecting my ability to trust and see the truth. It's a disease that doesn't just hurt you physically, it affects how you think and feel, too."

Knots form in Cole's throat as he tells me what happens next. "I walked over to a crucifix that's hanging in our house and I saw it different

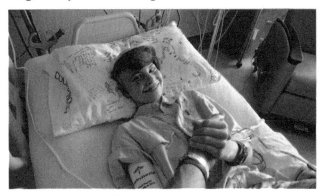

Cole during his cancer treatment.

51

than I ever had before. As a believer, I know Jesus suffered. It was ingrained in me by my parents when I was young. So in that moment, I *chose* to suffer – like Him. Because His plan is perfect. Ever since I accepted that, cancer hasn't had the same type of power over me."

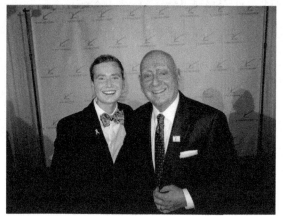

Cole with Dick at one of the many galas he has attended.

Cole is 22 years old now and since I've known him at age 14 he's helped teach me this invaluable lesson that not only applies to fighting cancer but any battle in life: Once you break free from the power grip that your own suffering can have over you – and we all have our different pathways of how we get to that destination, I know – then that's when one's purpose can start to crystalize.

Cole has helped me realize that suffering is as purposeful as it is unfair.

That's a difficult concept for me to take in at 84 years old. Cole figured it out when he was 12.

Lord knows I questioned my own diagnoses – in my first major bout with cancer in 2021-22 and then again when it took away my voice in 2023. At first I thought my life's purpose of helping these kids was being taken from me. None of it made sense to me then. I had negative thoughts when my body would be completely broken down from all the treatments.

Your mental approach is so vital when you're going through those dark moments. But it's not always easy to think positive and have faith. As Cole mentioned, so much of how cancer can break us is based on what it takes away. It took away his friends, his ability to play soccer, normalcy. For me, the worst part of my cancer battles was cancer taking away my voice.

The lymphoma in 2021 coincided with dysplasia of my vocal cords, which is a condition that put me on vocal-cord rest for several months in 2022. It officially became cancer in the summer of 2023. Altogether, those two bouts equated to seven of the worst months of my life being unable to speak to others.

Cole's message to me both times was right on par with Lorraine's: Not to let cancer and its aftermath steal my joy. Man, that's been the hardest thing to do because of what

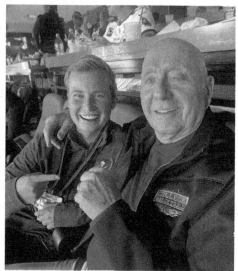

Cole and Dick at a Tampa Bay Buccaneers playoff game.

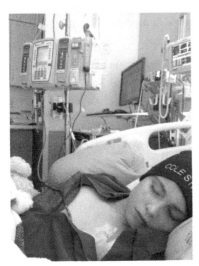
Cole during his cancer treatment.

my voice has provided me throughout my life as a broadcaster and philanthropist.

But it's been in young heroes like Cole that I've found my resolve. Instead of calling donors, I'll text. Instead of speaking out in public, I'll use a white board to express myself.

"We were all shocked when you got sick but we were praying for you every step of the way," Cole tells me. "I could tell the hardest part for you was not being able to speak for us. I remember feeling myself, 'Why Him? He's doing so much for our cause.' But then I remembered what we talk about with cancer not discriminating against anyone. I then thought about how you've changed since you had cancer and now you have so much more knowledge about the treatments we go through. If anything, it's made you want to fight for us even more."

Cole's spot on. My purpose to help kids has only been strengthened through my own experience.

But I'm no starting pitcher in this fight, I'm more like a relief pitcher in the seventh inning. These kids have already done all the grunt work on the cancer mound.

At the end of the day, I know my battle's still different. I got punched in the mouth by cancer after having lived a blessed life – deep into my fourth quarter. For these kids, though, their ability to rebound after fighting cancer in their first quarter is the stuff of true champions. Cole's a telltale example of this resurgence, now a senior at the University of South Florida and an intern for the Tampa Bay Buccaneers.

It's a misconception that once your treatment is done, you go back to living a regular life. That's totally untrue. In this new life that I've been living since being cancer free at 14, I always try to look towards the positives instead of the negatives.

- Cole Eicher

"It's a misconception that once your treatment is done, you go back to living a regular life," Cole says. "That's totally untrue. In this new life that I've been living since being cancer free at 13, I always try to look towards the positives instead of the negatives."

It certainly can feel like a whole new life in those first stages of recovery.

You see, I don't think I'm the only cancer survivor to feel this: That when you battle cancer, with all the tubes and bloodwork and needles, even if you become cancer-free, it's impossible to stay the same afterward. As Cole says, "There's no back to normal. It's a new normal."

Cole's new normal is two-pronged. He hasn't been the same on both a physical and emotional front.

From a physical perspective, Cole says: "Every day, I'm reminded of the effects from what I went through. The devastating long-term effects on kids aren't talked about enough. A lot of us are growing and not completely stable when we're being hit harder and harder with chemotherapy used for adults. It's a misconception that if you create a drug for adults, then you can just use it on kids – that childhood cancer can be treated just like adulthood cancer. It doesn't work that way."

That's why treatment plans, specifically catered to kids, are so important. Cole says his treatment plan proved to be a driving force in helping him battle against cancer.

"A good treatment plan is your best way to fight back," Cole says. "But I realize that there are so many pediatric cancers that don't have treatment plans. Some are just told you have six months to live."

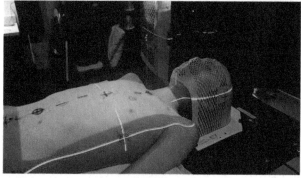

Cole during his cancer treatment.

Cole's treatment plan – it's even extended into his cancer-free adulthood – is all possible because of research. Here's how: When he was being treated for brain cancer, he underwent genetic testing that determined he would eventually need to address polyps that could've caused another type of cancer – colon cancer. Sure enough, the genetic testing was right and at 15 years old, in remission from brain cancer, Cole was able to have the polyps identified with just enough time to fend off colon cancer. He also was old enough at the time that a renowned surgeon at Tampa General Hospital was able to perform a surgery that thankfully kept Cole from having to have a colostomy bag the rest of his life.

Again, all because of research, doctors had the foresight to have him genetically tested. "I knew parents who lost their kids to colon cancer because it wasn't detected," his mother, Laura says.

"What's helped Cole on his journey is he's been able to trust in his treatment plans and lean on his faith. Even when we rolled him into brain surgery and he'd be all by himself with the doctors, he knew he wasn't alone because he had his faith in God."

Cole's continued to have ripple effects from his brain cancer battle and evasion of colon cancer. When I was visiting him at a Tampa Bay Buccaneers game – he's interned there for the past two summers under Chief Operations Officer Brian Ford – he told me a tumor had grown near his colon as a side effect of the surgery he underwent at 15. I was stunned, but thankfully realized that the tumor wasn't cancerous and that there's a new drug awaiting FDA approval that can help shrink the tumor.

Right when you think one kid can't go through enough, there's yet another adversity dropped on him.

The research is why he's with us today, though, make no mistake.

"When I go to the galas every year," Cole tells me, "it might sound cliché but the thing that I love to do is thank people. Whether it's $100 dollars or $10,000 dollars being donated, that money goes to research plans that saved my life and can potentially save other kids' lives."

FACT:
One in every 260 kids are diagnosed with cancer before turning 20.
- American Cancer Society

Like Sadie Keller, Cole also speaks to Congress to build awareness for legislatures to fund pediatric cancer research. He'll press them to treat it like the national priority it is. He'll talk about his story and apply it to jarring statistics like the fact that one in every 260 kids are diagnosed with cancer before turning 20 or that cancer is the No. 1 disease-related cause of death for children ages 1-19.

"I tell them I've been to countless funerals of my friends for a kid my age, that they're why I'm speaking to them," Cole says of being before Congress. "They eventually get it. But it's sort of like, you don't believe it until you see it."

That seeing-is-believing factor is exactly why for so long I've chosen to have my All-Courageous Team of kids out front at fundraiser events. They're the face of this movement. I just try to play pass-first point guard and get them that assist, baby.

"One of Cole's sayings has been, 'Everyone can do something,' " Laura says. "He'd go to speak to pro sports teams in the Tampa area – mainly the Tampa Rowdies soccer team – and ask the athletes, 'What are you doing for others outside of yourself?' Because once you know about something like childhood cancer, once you really see it, you can't look the other way."

Cole recalls that right after he was diagnosed, he was taken aback when he walked into Johns Hopkins All Children's Hospital in St. Petersburg and saw kids on tricycles with their chemo bags and realized that many of the parents weren't able to even be there because they had to work to pay for their kids' treatments.

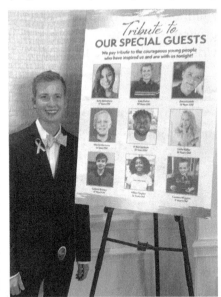

Cole with the Courageous Kids display at the gala.

"Before then, I just thought cancer was something that happened to adults. I realized then and there that this awareness piece about kids outside of the hospital was not there," Cole says. "I could feel the overall support side with childhood cancer lacking so I immediately wanted to help."

That's when Cole started to learn more about the value of research and treatment plans. Determined to help in any way he could on his level, he felt a calling to be a speaker for these kids.

Cole was a highly successful soccer player way back before he was diagnosed. (His top memory is playing with his U12 soccer team against Bayern Munich in Germany.) His experience as a midfielder gave him a natural inclination to help others. Then factor in that he had done some modeling and acting – and his purpose started to take shape.

An emotional Laura recalls: "Cole came to me and said, 'Mom, nobody ever told me about kids having cancer. Why isn't it being talked about, why aren't there kids helping kids?' He then goes, 'I'm not afraid to speak to adults about hard topics. God's been training me for this. I'm gonna be their voice.' "

And their voice he has become.

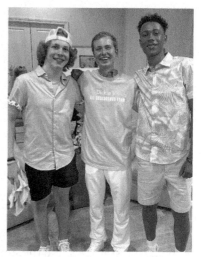

Weston Hermann, Cole, and Jayden Spencer.

He's now a key spokesperson and founder of the American Cancer Society's "Gold Together" for childhood cancer initiative in which funds raised are dedicated to childhood cancer research and support programs. During Cole's battle in his early teens, his grade school friends wore "COLE STRONG" rubber wristbands that cited Jeremiah 29:11. The bible verse states that the Lord has "plans to prosper you and not harm you, plans to give you hope and a future."

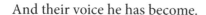

Now he's sharing that hope with everyone he can touch.

It brings me back to what most impressed me about Cole when I first met him: He felt as though there wasn't enough being done for kids, so he helped raise funds to create a Teen Lounge at All-Children's Hospital in St. Petersburg, Florida. That's where teens could play games, relax, and read magazines. It could be a safe haven from all the treatment, a place to connect with other battlers, a place where nurses and parents are asked to stay outside the doors.

In my first chapter, I told you the story of Tony Colton. Cole and Tony became good buds, with Tony a little older. What's so touching to me is that the same lounge Cole helped build was where Tony and his family ended up going for refuge in the months and weeks before he passed.

"Tony's mom texted me and said we broke the record for how many people can fit in that room," Laura says. "That made us feel so good, that something Cole created could give him and his family a little joy."

As Lorraine has cautioned me, joy is one emotion that can be robbed as much as any when you have a cancer story – during a fight, and after it. Survivor's guilt is an experience many of these kids can have. Someone like Cole can say, "Why Tony and not me, God?" But the way I see it, that's just an extension of those original negative thoughts that come when cancer brings us to our knees.

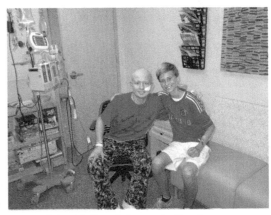

Cole with Tony Colton at the Teen Lounge.

The winning ingredient in the recipe is keeping your joy, as Cole so often says.

"That's why when you rang the bell to be cancer-free (the first time in 2022) and started dancing, it inspired all of us," Cole tells me. "We could see cancer wasn't going to steal your joy."

Inspiring is the least I can do to return the favor. I learned from the best, Cole.

Cole volunteers for the American Cancer Society and is a spokesman for the "Gold Together" campaign.

To donate to the V Foundation,
Dick Vitale Pediatric Cancer Research Fund,
please scan this code.

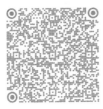

Chapter

Seven

Tears of Strength

with the Cannon Wiggins Family

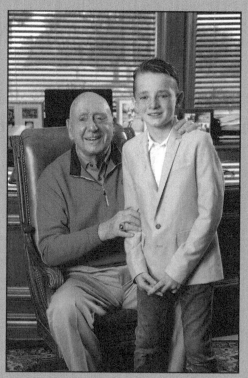

"If you've ever watched a kid fight cancer,
it'll change your life forever."
- Michael Wiggins

Tears drip down the face of 12-year-old Cannon Wiggins.

I'm asking him about what he remembers from his torturous battle with cancer that started before he was two.

"It was super hard," he says. "You…don't really ever get past it."

The tears are his body's response to words like *chemotherapy*, *radiation* and *stem cell treatment*. He is seven years in remission, but his bout with cancer has left him with a post-traumatic reaction, as if from a war.

Think about that for a second. A war. That's what these kids experience, with their parents fighting beside them, yet unable to fight it *for* them.

Cannon's as brave a warrior as they come, the kind of warrior who went through 106 consecutive hours of drip chemotherapy in the bag and survived. All so he could have a stem-cell transplant next. That type of stat line shows *Awesome* courage. With a Capital A.

That palpable sense of courage is always in the room with Cannon. He sits down for an interview to talk about this book and waves his Mom and Dad off to speak for himself. But before we converse about this difficult subject, he goes to his room to get a protective red robe. I realize halfway through the conversation that the robe helps disguise his tears better.

It's hard to convince a 12-year-old boy in the thick of middle school that it's okay to cry. That's where I try to lead by example. I cry about kids like him all the time. I hope they see that if an 84-year-old man can cry his eyes out, they can too.

> *Cannon's as brave a warrior as they come, the kind of warrior who went through 106 consecutive hours of drip chemotherapy in the bag and survived. …That type of stat line shows Awesome courage. With a Capital A.*
>
> *- Dick Vitale*

Jimmy V told us all before he left: "If you laugh, you think, and you cry, that's a full day. That's a heck of a day. You do that seven days a week, you're going to have something special."

Jimmy embraced tears as strength, and all I can see when these kids like Cannon shed their own tears is absolute strength.

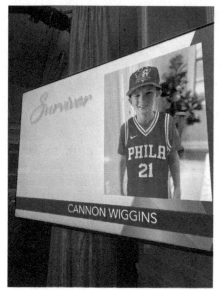

Cannon on the All-Courageous Team.

Cannon's one of the superstars on the All-Courageous Team of kids that I assemble every year for my gala. I've had the privilege in my life of establishing relationships with some of the most talented athletes, coaches and media members in sports history. All of these sports megastars rise to their feet when kids like Cannon are honored on the stage.

His cancer story is one of perseverance and beating the odds – literally.

My first encounter with the Wiggins family was through an event I did with former San Francisco Giants catcher Buster Posey. At the 2016 fundraiser, Buster introduced Cannon's father, Michael Wiggins, to say a few words. During his speech, Michael opened up about the type of adult chemotherapy, cisplatin, that little Cannon would have to endure to survive. The medicine is so toxic that he and Melissa had to sign papers acknowledging their son would likely lose hearing.

Let that sink in. As a parent, you're signing on to an attempt to save your son's life while simultaneously signing on for a future disability. That's outrageously unfair.

"In the journey that we went on with Cannon, not one time was he treated with a drug that's specifically approved and designed for children," Michael says. "He was treated with adult forms the whole time, starting at two years old. That's so unjust. I saw this kid throw up more than I have in my entire adult life before he was even two years old.

"If you've ever watched a kid fight cancer, it'll change your life forever."

Melissa, Cannon's mother, remembers the world stopping. She tells me the story of being 38 weeks pregnant with twins and being initially upset that then-20-month-old Cannon would have to wear a cast on his leg for a minor injury. Then she got the dreaded call from an oncologist and heard *neuroblastoma* come out of his mouth for the first time.

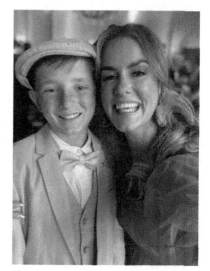

Cannon with his mom, Melissa.

"I had never heard of neuroblastoma, so I asked the doctor what it was," Melissa recalls, her own tears streaming. "He said it's a very aggressive form of pediatric cancer."

The doctor later explained Cannon's case was Stage IV, had spread to his hip, leg, and shoulder; and was high risk. At the time, neuroblastoma was the deadliest form of pediatric cancer.

"I felt like I had an elephant on my chest," Melissa says. "I couldn't breathe. I handed the phone to my husband. I said, 'You need to talk to the doctor.' I walked out of the room because I didn't want Cannon to see me upset."

These are the conversations that can debilitate you as a parent.

"I'm 14 years sober and was a few years sober at the time," Melissa shares. "I called my sponsor and that night I had a breakdown with her on the phone. I laid it all out there. Afterwards, that was it. I wasn't about to let my son fight through that alone."

FACT:
1 in 7 children diagnosed with cancer in the U.S. will not survive.
Overall, childhood cancer remains the most common cause of death by disease among children in the U.S.
– Children's Cancer Research Fund

Michael and Melissa tell me they had to get "gritty" for little Cannon, who went through treatments all across the country from Orlando to New York to Gainesville to Grand Rapids to Philadelphia. At the time, the best way to treat neuroblastoma was an onslaught approach: Throw everything at the cancer from chemo to radiation to stem-cell treatment – again, all the adult kinds. No matter how grueling it is on the child, doctors told the Wiggins family a more conservative approach could risk a relapse. And, at the time, the survivor rate after a relapse was terrible.

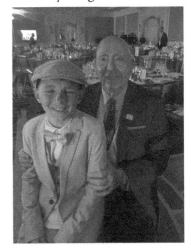

"Michael and I shifted from, 'This is so traumatic, what can we do?' to 'Okay, we've got to figure things out and really push into our resilience skills,' " Melissa says.

For so many parents thrust into such a circumstance, once the acceptance part kicks in, all they need is a sliver of hope to switch into warrior mode.

"When Melissa left the room and I talked to the oncologist in that initial visit," Michael recalls, "he basically told me Cannon's survival rate was 50/50."

Dick with Cannon at the gala.

Can you imagine? For these unbelievably strong families, cancer sadly becomes a game of odds.

Cannon was not yet two and his chances of survival hinged on what decisions his parents made, which regimen they decided on for Cannon's treatment.

"To this day," Michael says, "there are two major paths you can take for treatment of neuroblastoma because there hasn't been enough research. One is sponsored by Sloan Kettering, the other by Children's Oncology Group, both with some successful (survivor) rates. Once you choose as a family to go down a certain path, if it doesn't work and the child is not responding, with no tumor shrinkage, you can't just jump over to the other paths."

That horrific either-or choice is one of many byproducts from there not being enough research or treatment avenues for children battling cancer.

"We've seen other parents lose their child after going down a certain path," Michael continues. "So, not only do you lose your child in that case. But you have to live the rest of your life, thinking, 'I wonder if I should've taken the other path? Did I make the right choice?' The funds for clinical trials may not save a child's life, but they at least can help secure one path for treatment so families don't have to live in that type of misery."

From a macro perspective, kids with cancer need medicines and procedures specifically catered to them, and not to adults. From a micro perspective, as the Wiggins family can attest, better research provides more needed clarity on which specific path to take.

FACT:
Neuroblastoma is a rare type of childhood cancer, currently the third most common behind leukemia and brain tumors, with 75 percent of patients diagnosed by age 5. There are 12 major types of childhood cancers and over 100 subtypes.
– Children's Cancer Research Fund

"Making those choices is really hard when it's your kid's life on the line," Melissa recalls. "You almost have to dissociate from it when you're trying to make a really smart choice."

Thank God Melissa trusted her "momma gut" as she tells me of a decision with a clinical trial in Michigan that saved Cannon's life.

The same doctor who diagnosed Cannon originally told Michael and Melissa they were "idiots" if they went through with a trial for a drug called difluoromethylornithine (DFMO).

"A lot of doctors didn't agree with what we did for Cannon," Melissa says. "But we did so much research and knew this was what we had to do."

Neuroblastoma is a type of pediatric cancer, like so many, where the goal is No Evidence of Disease (NED). Doctors won't use words like "cured" or even "cancer-free" because of the cancer's ability to return in aggressive fashion. The hardest part isn't getting to that NED point so much as it is to stay there. That's why Michael and Melissa opted to go for the clinical trial for Cannon, knowing that the DFMO treatment had strong signs of stopping the genes from turning back so that the cancer cells ultimately won't return.

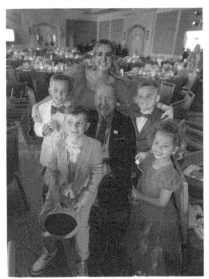

Dick with Cannon, mom Melissa, and his siblings at the gala.

Fast forward to today and DFMO is the leading form of treatment for neuroblastoma, based on the patient. Boy, was Melissa right. The momma gut, baby, coming up clutch.

Michael and Melissa knew a family whose daughter was two years older than Cannon and they weren't able to use DFMO. Their daughter died this past summer.

"Most of the kids who were diagnosed with Cannon aren't here anymore," Melissa says, eyes moist.

Michael remembers Cannon's most dangerous surgery where the surgeon stood for 13 hours straight to remove the cancer. Beforehand the surgeon said there was a 2/10 chance he could remove it all while keeping little Cannon alive.

Cannon beat the odds.

That trauma from all the percentages doesn't go away, even after the battle's over. Because you're so close to the other side.

I still have a deeply meaningful text saved from Michael just imagining being on the other side of the coin. He messaged and pleaded in 2017, "Please, Dickie V and Lorraine, don't stop fighting for kids like my son so that my wife and I are not one of seven (cancer-affected) parents who have to dress up to go to the funeral of their child. I can't even imagine."

As Michael wrote that, he was in a gripping juxtaposition thinking about another father he knew who that very day was putting on his best suit to bury his child.

"I've been to several funerals myself with kids we know from this disease," Michael says. "It's just heartbreaking and infuriating at the same time."

It shouldn't ever have to come to 50/50 decisions. We're making strides, getting better, at least. I'm happy to tell you that as I write, kids can survive more frequently after a relapse. The odds have improved.

Nowadays, Cannon is living that normal kid life, avidly playing basketball and football, gaming on Roblox and Fortnite, and going down waterslides at waterparks. He has to wear a hearing aid and is smaller than most boys for his age. These are two of the side effects from all the chemo and radiation his body

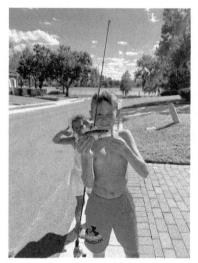

Cannon and a big catch!

endured. And he has to take one shot every night. Otherwise, he's living free from the nemesis that tortured the first part of his life.

When I ask him about how his life is different with cancer in the rear-view mirror, he tells me, "I get to have fun now. Cancer took away the fun."

That's so much of the tragedy right there. This ruthless disease robs kids of having the fun they deserve because they're constantly in next-treatment or life-or-death mode. That leaves psychological scars as much as it does physical.

Don't forget the siblings. They suffer, too. Michael had to miss the birth of twins Arran and Gray because he was in a hospital room 100 yards away with Cannon going through chemotherapy.

Cannon and his twin brothers are close in age, less than two years apart, so that brotherly dynamic becomes a huge factor in the healing process. "I really think," Melissa says, "that Cannon is in part alive because of Arran and Gray. Without them, Cannon wouldn't have been fighting as hard as he did. Because he saw them and wanted to play with them at 2, 3, 4 and 5 years old. They were back then and are now three best little buddies."

Gray says he'd like to go onstage at my galas, "but I don't want to get those shots that (Cannon) has to get."

Melissa says Gray and Arran sometimes get jealous when Cannon gets gifts, like a Tom Brady-signed jersey: "The twins are like, 'Wait, I love those things, too.'"

It's a credit to the Wiggins that they do their best to balance Cannon's bravery while also keeping the spotlight on all their children, including 25-year-old daughter Oliva, and 6-year-old daughter, Charlie.

The family has come to my galas for the last six years, recently bringing the entire family. That's where Cannon loves the "VIP" treatment we try to give youngsters and their families. His brothers love that they can order six Shirley Temples at a time.

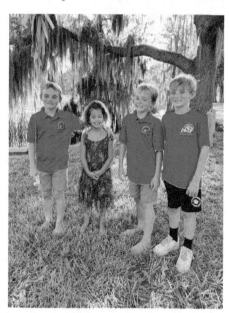

Cannon with his siblings.

The day after last year's gala, I saw the three boys throwing around the football at a gathering in my backyard. It's in those moments that I see two stories: One story of three brothers having a blast. The other of a kid who went through hell and who is finally getting his fun back.

"The thing I admire about Cannon the most is how he survived," Arran says. "I don't like cancer because it scares me. When you know someone who survived, you're pretty lucky."

Luck shouldn't come down to 50/50, or worse. We're working to change that. Count on it, Cannon.

Michael and Melissa Wiggins raise money for childhood cancer with their foundation, cannonballkidscancer.org. To date, CKc has raised more than $3 million and created 687 treatment options for children whose only other alternative was hospice.

Melissa Wiggins' new book chronicling her family's journey, UnFollow: Question EVERYTHING With Excitement, is available on Amazon.

To donate to the V Foundation,
Dick Vitale Pediatric Cancer Research Fund,
please scan this code.

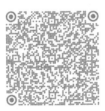

Chapter Eight

Post-Traumatic Resurgence

with the Enzo Grande Family

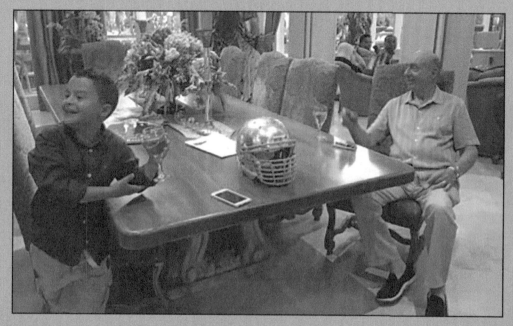

"The mental health part of it isn't talked about enough. ...There's not really any support out there for families after the fact or even 5-10 years down the road. The support is out there during the fight."
- Vince Grande

Opening a family-run Italian restaurant can come with its fair share of stress. But Enzo Grande and his family know a thing or two about managing family stress.

The brand-new business challenges hardly compare to the life-and-death stress that the family faced when Enzo battled leukemia. He's 16 now; he was 3 ½ when he was diagnosed. The following four years were, as his mother puts it, "hell on earth."

And now, a lifetime later, Enzo plays high school football and waits tables at the family restaurant in Ponte Vedra, Florida. Vincenzo's Cucina, which opened its doors this year, serves an assortment of Italian and American dishes – including a burger named after me! – and of course, mouth-watering pastas and flatbreads. From one paison to another, you might say it's a little slice of heaven.

"I've been so proud to see my Mom and Dad and all of us working as a team," Enzo says. "There's been stress that comes along with it, but it's been amazing to actually see it go well and to see the smiles on my parents' faces."

Make no mistake, this is the good kind of stress. The triumphant kind, if you will. The future looks bright, even if sometimes flashes from the past intrude on the present.

"I went to put on black latex gloves to cook something at the restaurant," Enzo's mother, Elaine, says. "Then it all came back and hit me so hard. I hadn't put on gloves like that since I was giving Enzo chemo treatment. He hated those needles more than anything and had to get at least one shot a day."

The Grande family is suffering from post-traumatic stress, just like so many cancer-stricken families in the aftermath following years of treatment.

"Whenever he coughs or sneezes, we look at each other," Enzo's father, Vince, says. "Even if it's just a cold, we associate it with, 'Oh my god we have to go through it again.'"

Enzo hates needles to this day. He has ongoing struggles with anxiety. "I'll worry about my health a lot and if I'm allergic to anything," he says. "Sometimes I just worry and worry about the worst-case thing happening."

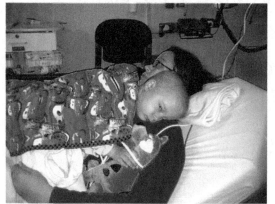
Enzo with his mom, Elaine, in his cancer fight.

Because Enzo is allergic to most pain medications, including morphine, Vince and Elaine had to hold their son in their arms while they rocked him to sleep for procedures.

"At one point during his chemotherapy, we had to stop treatment because he was turning yellow and doctors worried he may have a second cancer," Vince says. "You cannot unsee these things."

"There were these moments that just stay with you forever," Elaine says. "We had to watch him go through these procedures where he was laying there lifeless. ...I still have a lot of bitterness and anger for all he went through, how unfair it was for him. Sooner or later, I'll be able to be grateful he's healthy, playing football now. But it's still too close to the storm."

Enzo's battle – or storm, as Elaine calls it – involved four years of chemotherapy, 18 spinal taps, 20 blood transfusions, and one liver disorder. It left the Grandes to pick up the pieces of debris, simply trying to rebuild a sense of normalcy in the aftermath. The family showed great strength during Enzo's cancer fight – and after it, too.

"The mental-health part of it isn't talked about enough," Vince tells me. "We didn't have the funds to do therapy, there's not really any support out there for families after the fact or even five-to-10 years down the road. The support is out there during the fight.

"For four years, everything was about keeping our son alive. Elaine had a part-time job at night when she wasn't being a full-time nurse to Enzo. I worked two jobs just to make ends meet."

The Grande family followed the playbook of so many families like them: Doing anything at any cost to save your child. They moved five times in three years, at times living in a one-bedroom apartment with Enzo and his twin sister, Larissa. Elaine says Larissa has been Enzo's biggest supporter through the years, with the bond between the twins "unbreakable" – even when the family's stability felt broken in half at times.

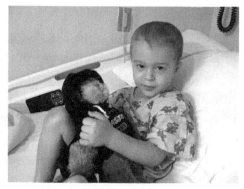
Enzo in his cancer fight.

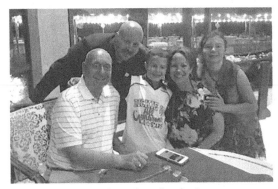

The Grandes with Dick at his home.

"Sometimes you have negative 20 dollars in your checking account and your child wants a toy," Vince says. "There's no real support for that. You can't always do it financially because cancer breaks families' entire world."

Vince is so right. Yes, of course we need dollars to help oncologists come up with cures and safer treatments catered to kids. But the emotional and financial burdens that come in the direct aftermath of a family fighting cancer are important, too. That's why seeing the Grandes in their element, with their brand-new restaurant, brings me so much joy. Because I can see what they went through – what they're still going through – to get to this point. Their resurgence is sensational, baby.

But other families aren't so lucky. Enzo will be the first to tell you of how his family has been "blessed" along the uphill road to recovery. I got them in touch with Stephanie McMahon, former co-CEO of WWE. (She attended my gala in 2016 and spearheaded major donations to it over the years.) McMahon showcased the Grande family on the TV show, *Undercover Boss*, when Enzo was 9. And, oh boy, you can see Enzo's star power in the video clips.

Enzo's room nowadays is like a mini sports museum. There are helmets, balls, signed photos, and all manner of memorabilia from my galas over the years – including an autograph with a prayer from Clemson football coach Dabo Swinney. Most meaningfully, he has a picture of the two of us on his nightstand.

I get emotional when I hear Vince and Elaine tell me Enzo aspires to be a TV personality like me. It means so much to hear Enzo speak about his goals and desires. His personality is dynamic and his love for sports is special. He's a telltale example of a kid who hasn't let cancer stop him from chasing his dreams. In fact, I think his arduous road has propelled him to chase them even more.

He's close with my ESPN colleagues Kevin Negandhi and Scott Van Pelt, two anchors who are the best in the business. He also had a relationship with the late Stuart Scott. He even emulates Stuart's "Boo-yah" charisma. These mentors all have

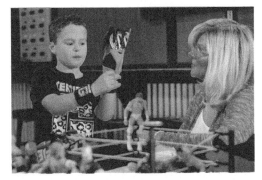

Enzo with Stephanie McMahon for Undercover Boss.

seen what I've seen in this youngster: Greatness. Let me tell you, my friends, Enzo Grande will be a big winner in the game of life with his desire and determination. Much of that credit goes to his loving parents who, like many in this book, fought tooth and nail to save their child's life.

Enzo calls me "Uncle Dick" and pays me one of the most special compliments when he says he wants to be like me – and not just as a broadcaster: "I want to be like you in how you fight against pediatric cancer."

Little does Enzo know he's already a little like me in that way as a cancer spokesman. He mentors kids from Australia and Hawaii who are battling cancer. He started "Enzo's Smackdown to Cancer," a wrestling-themed toy drive for cancer patients near his home in St. Augustine, Fla. He's truly embraced his role from a small age.

"I tell Enzo," Vince says, "God chose you to be an apostle, to stay here so that you can continue and help."

Enzo tells me that he understands why I took the baton from Jimmy V all those years ago. And I tell Enzo there is no *Dick Vitale vs. Cancer* if Jimmy didn't show me – and the world – what fighting is all about.

> *I tell Enzo, 'God chose you to be an apostle, to stay here so that you can continue and help.'*
>
> *- Vince Grande*

"He's probably looking down from heaven and thinking, 'How is Dick doing all this?' He started it and now you're out here finishing it," Enzo says.

I am fighting to finish what Jimmy V started. As I'm writing this book, it's been 30 years since his passing and I feel as committed as ever to take his advice.

As I underwent radiation treatment in late 2023 – and suffered its side effects – Jimmy's words echoed in my head: "I always have to think about what's important in life to me. There are these three things: Where you started, where you are, and where you're going to be."

When I see Enzo and his family, I see where they started – in the battle for his life. I see where they are now – on the other side, having opened *Vincenzo's Cucina*. And I see where they're going – a clear runway for Enzo to keep chasing his dreams.

The Grande family is Italian, like Jimmy V and me. "Italians help Italians," says Vince. "We like to hug and be passionate." He's certainly right about that.

That burger named after me will have all proceeds go to the V Foundation. That's just incredible. I am moved beyond words.

Enzo with Dick at the gala.

Vince and Elaine are torn on the notion that everything happens for a reason. Enzo suffered tremendously, and so did they. "I wouldn't wish what we went through on anyone," Elaine says. Then again, they say they wouldn't change anything either. Their son's suffering has led him to where he is now – a determined teen set out to help rid the world of cancer.

Enzo carries emotional scars that have shaped him into who he is today. Recently he wrote on TikTok:

I was always smiling as a kid but little Enzo didn't know what was coming.

My family and I were at Disney and we went to see Cars, *the movie. For some reason, I was really tired all the time and got really sick.*

Then we went to the hospital and no one knew what I had. We went to Orlando to go to a hospital there and they told my family something that would change our lives forever: I had cancer.

The memories fade. But the emotions are less erasable. Vince and Elaine say they're still haunted by some of the things they saw at Children's Hospital of Philadelphia.

Fact:
30-45 percent of parents and siblings and 15-20 percent of childhood cancer survivors
experience severe symptoms of post-traumatic stress several years after treatment has ended.
- Children's Hospital of Philadelphia

"When you go into the hospital waiting room and see kids who are grey and shaking from all the radiation and chemo, you can't forget that hopelessness and powerlessness," Elaine says. "It's the sick of the sick in there. To this day, it felt like hell on Earth."

The Grandes credit Enzo's nurses over the years as being the angels in that inferno – guiding their child to be alive and well today. It's the rainbow after the storm. Elaine hopes someday she can see its colors. "I'm just not there yet," she says.

Enzo is helping her gradually to see the rainbow. He posted a photo of himself on TikTok that shows him when he learned he was cancer-free. The caption said it all.

I was so excited I got to ring the bell. It was a journey. I know I can't remember a lot from when I was a kid, but I don't know how 'little me' did what I did. After this, I was thinking I want to help kids with cancer from now on.

My family is amazing. I don't know where I'd be without them.

So yeah, I survived cancer but now I need to help kids with cancer so the job's not finished.

I can't ask for a better life right now.

Vincenzo's is located in Ponte Vedra, Florida, in St. John's County.
Portions of the proceeds from items on the menu go to the V Foundation.

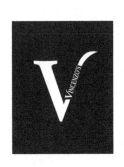

Chapter Nine
Bonded for Life

with the Katelyne Ballesteros Family

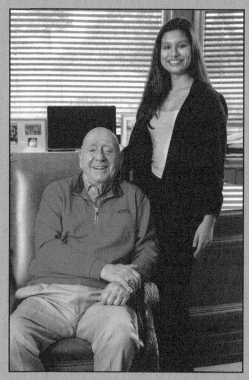

"Whatever I do, it will be to help children in some way."
- Katelyne Ballesteros

Katelyne Ballesteros was 12 at the time. She had acute leukemia and needed chemotherapy – fast. If she waited even a week, oncologists told her they may not be able to kill the cancer quickly enough for her to live.

That's when her doctors gave Katelyne and her family a terrible choice: Should she have the chemo immediately? Or did she want to save her eggs first so that she might someday have biological children of her own?

"It came down to my life or my future kids' lives," Katelyne tells me, the tears dripping down. "They told me the adult chemo I was putting in my body would eliminate my ability to have children."

In that moment, Katelyne and her mother, Maria Moraites, and stepfather, John Moraites, chose not to put her life at risk by waiting. It was the right decision. Yet a decision no child should ever have to make.

"As I got older and realized I wanted kids at some point, then you start to feel the loss," Katelyne says. "It just makes me sad. I was young and reacted off of instinct – rationally. ...I was 12 years old and was just thinking about trying to stay alive."

And the rest of us think we have problems?

Adoption is an option down the road perhaps. But it's expensive and Katelyne admits she's not past the loss tied to having children of her own.

"People will say to me, 'It's okay because there are miracles and other ways to have a baby,'" Katelyne says. "The reality for me is that it's not okay. For me personally, I see pregnancy as a beautiful thing where it bonds you with a child. Cancer took that from me forever.

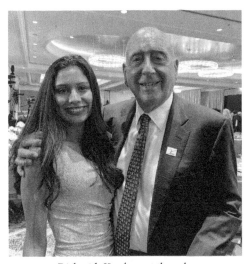

Dick with Katelyne at the gala.

"We don't think about the lifelong complications or side-effects until we get over the bridge."

Katelyne's over that cancer bridge now and living her life to the fullest despite the side effects that also include a heart condition. She's 20 and studying at Hillsborough Community College in Florida with plans to be an ultrasound nurse. What could be more fitting than that?

"When I work with patients, in the future, I will have knowledge first-hand of what they may be going through from all my treatments when I was younger," Katelyne says. "I can relate to them, help them to not feel alone. Because sometimes the doctors have to remain super professional and it's so important that kids are feeling empathy in those scenarios where they're fighting for their life and when they've lost all normalcy."

Katelyne feels compassion for patients she hasn't even met yet. That's a sample size of what she will bring to the medical field. It will be meaningful, let me tell you. Those moments alone in the hospital when your family leaves, or is resting, that's when a nurse warmly checking in on you can mean the world. And she knows that as well as anyone. She will be a natural – a PTP-er of a nurse. Trust me.

She's working as a nanny while going to college, which figures. "I've always known I love kids and being around them," she says. "Whatever I do, it will be to help children in some way."

When she was a child herself, she used to nickname her nurses after Disney princesses. Belle from *Beauty and the Beast*. Aurora from *Sleeping Beauty*. Cinderella from *Cinderella*. And on and on. Katelyne found ways to stay in her imagination because her reality was no fairy tale.

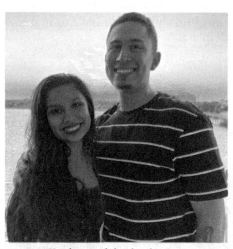

Katelyne with her brother Luis.

At one point her treatment included many aggressive cycles of chemotherapy. Each cycle lasted a week or more. Through it all, she offered the utmost respect to the team treating her. It's a lesson for us all. It's not just your family members who are in your corner. It's also the doctors, the nurses, the hospital workers. Everyone. They are, after all, playing a huge part in trying to save your life.

Still, family is the first line of defense. Katelyne knows this firsthand. Her brother, Luis, then 19, was the donor for a bone-marrow transplant. She had a B+ blood type beforehand and that prompted Katelyne's mantra, her battle cry, in her fight against cancer: "Be positive!" Her brother had an A+ blood type and now they both have A+ blood types since the transplant. "I consider him my twin now," Katelyne says.

Luis was in the U.S. Navy and stationed in Tokyo at the time. The fact that she didn't have to wait on a donor list to find a match probably saved her life. Thankfully, Luis's Navy schedule allowed him to come home and give his little sister the gift of life.

It brought us closer and gave us a stronger bond. It's something I'll cherish forever.

- Katelyne Ballesteros on her brother, Luis, when he became a donor for a bone-marrow transplant that saved her life.

"If there wasn't a match, I would have gone on the national list," she says. "I still remember the FaceTime call when my brother told me it was going to be him. I just had a dream where God told me someone would come to help save me. I just had no idea it would actually be my brother.

"I'll always feel like, 'How could I repay him?' It brought us closer and gave us a stronger bond. It's something I'll cherish forever."

Luis pushes back at such hero talk: "When I was a match and they asked if I was willing to donate, it was an easy decision – without a doubt. I was like, 'Of course!' Who wouldn't do that?"

Luis says he tries not to remember too much from his sister's cancer fight. But some things stay etched in memory.

"When they cut her hair off and we saw her little bald head, that was hard because it made it real," Luis says. "I was in shock, it felt like I was in a movie, so you don't know how to react. I remember eventually rubbing her head and trying to make light of it to take the (tension) off."

Katelyne's mother, Maria, was nearly always at her bedside. On one of the few days her mother could not be there, Katelyne had her only adverse reaction to chemo: She had a fever and hallucinated.

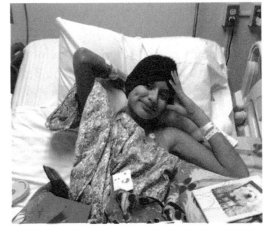

Katelyne in her cancer treatment.

"That was so scary," Katelyne says. "I remember feeling so safe with my mother, she was always there for me and never cried. So, the one time she wasn't there, it was like my body had to respond to it. I can't imagine getting through everything without my mother's help."

Katelyne's cancer was diagnosed after she moved from Chicago to Tampa Bay when her mother married stepfather John. The family was within walking distance of the hospital where Katelyne received her treatments, which was nice. But her birth father was still in Chicago, which was hard.

Then, almost exactly a year after Katelyne rang the bell, her father was diagnosed with stomach cancer. She got a final visit to see him in Chicago before he passed away, in 2018.

"I have anger towards cancer because of what it does to people, what it does to families," Katelyne says.

"I didn't have a childhood and it changed me as a person. No one knows how bad cancer is until it hits home."

Still, Katelyne tries to keep alive those special moments she had with her father before her cancer, and his, to honor their father-daughter bond.

"Nothing can change the love we have for each other," she says. "We used to watch telenovelas together and he always loved to eat. We'd also listen to music, he loved the band REO Speedwagon. He just loved to sing and would always do karaoke."

Katelyne feels compassion for patients she hasn't even met yet. That's a sample size of what she will bring to the medical field. She will be a natural – a PTP-er of a nurse. Trust me.

- Dick Vitale on Katelyne Ballesteros

Katelyne also lost her best friend to cancer. He came into her life because of their mutual interests and experiences, the biggest of which was their fight with cancer. Katelyne says it was "all the little things" outside of cancer that defined her special bond with Jayden Ojeda.

They met at a volleyball game of a mutual friend and hit it off immediately.

"Our friendship was truly unique, we instantly clicked," Katelyne says. "Our routine FaceTime calls became a cornerstone of our bond."

Among her most cherished memories with Jayden was a getaway to a beach house in Madeira Beach, alongside Jayden's mom, Alicia, and his sisters, Sacaria and Jena.

Such moments of respite are pivotal in a battle against cancer. They give you moments of peace that are otherwise robbed. And when you deal with cancer on a daily basis, you don't take anything for granted. The normal days become blessed days, especially if they're limited.

"That experience was surreal, like a beautiful dream," she recalls. "We immersed ourselves in the moment, free from worries. We soaked in the joy of playing games, sharing laughter, and enjoyed the sun and sand on the beach."

When times were tough, Jayden and Katelyne were there for each other. "We knew we could count on one another," she says. "We were there for each other whether we were stressed, scared or excited."

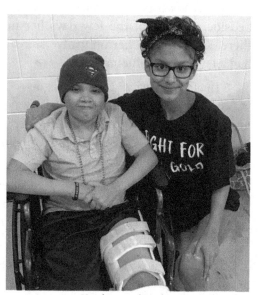
Katelyne and Jayden.

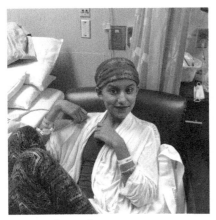

Katelyne in her cancer treatment.

Jayden was diagnosed on April 11, 2017, at the age of 12 with Osteosarcoma in his left tibia. "We never really talked about what our bond was, but everyone knew we were best friends from how we were around each other," Katelyne says.

Jayden fought a courageous battle for two and a half years before "gaining his angel wings" on his 15th birthday.

"I would cry myself to sleep sometimes," Katelyne says. "Like, why did I survive?"

Survivor's guilt can take you to a dark place. I know the feeling. Nowadays Katelyne uses the hole in her heart that is Jayden to tell his story alongside her own when she's speaking to cancer battlers in hospitals for charity work.

Katelyne carries Jayden's friendship and legacy with her in her heart, much as I carry the loss of Jimmy V in mine. It's not just a bond for life, as they say. "It's bonded forever," Katelyne says. The same could be said for her "twin" bond with Luis or her connection to her late father.

I still remember meeting Katelyne way back in 2016 shortly after her treatments ended. Her smile remains radiant every time I see her. Her family has showed me such warmth at my galas and at the post-party picnics at my house. I still have the letter Katelyne wrote me during my bout with lymphoma:

"Dear Mr. Vitale, I have been thinking about you and praying for you. You truly are inspirational, and I hope to pass on to you what you have taught me and many others. You are not alone! We are all in this together! Stay strong and positive. We love you."

Holy cow! I swear it's like the words inject you with a serum to heal in a time of need. She's right: We're never alone in this fight. We are all in this together. We are a true cancer-beating team, baby!

I feel humbled when she tells me what my cancer battle can mean to others. "We've always needed an ambassador for children's cancer because our stories can't be told without someone who can shine a light on our voice," she tells me. "Now we have a leader who knows exactly what we go through physically with treatments, the type of perseverance needed. Everything happens for a reason and I think you've gone through (cancer) so fewer people have to feel alone."

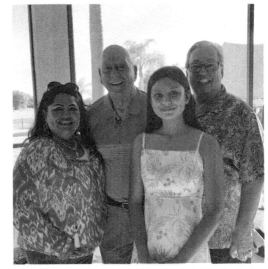

Dick with Katelyne and her family at the Vitale picnic.

In other words, I'm not just talking the talk anymore. I'm walking the walk. It's now empathy mixed with experience.

Katelyne calls me a guardian angel on her journey. It's fitting, I have to say, because she's returned the favor – and then some – with how she empowered me during my fight against vocal-cord cancer in 2023. I feel angel's wings of protection from this special girl.

During that voiceless battle I endured, she sent me a video. The message: Be positive, of course.

"I just wanted to let you know you're not alone in this battle," she says. "Your strength and courage inspire all of us. Be positive and focus on each small victory. You are loved and we believe in your ability to overcome. Keep fighting and know there are brighter days ahead. You've got this."

It's like she's already stepping into her future role – a life purpose, perhaps – as a nurse with knowhow in this worldwide cancer fight.

Which Disney princess of a nurse will Katelyne be someday? "That's up to someone else to decide," she says with a smile.

Maybe so, but this princess-to-be is already royalty to me.

To donate to the V Foundation,
Dick Vitale Pediatric Cancer Research Fund,
please scan this code.

Chapter Ten
Overcoming Depression
with the Coleton Korney Family

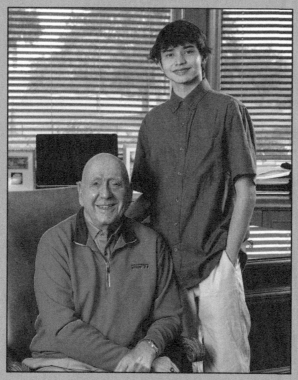

"You don't just walk away from cancer. It's not chicken pox. He's had all these bouts of depression and a lot of that stems from the fact that he's never going to be back to him."
- Danielle Korney on her son, Coleton

Halloween at a hospital happens in reverse.

The children can't go house to house, so the nurses go room to room, handing out candy to costumed kids. It's a way to make the most of a tough situation.

Art and Danielle Korney, self-described "dork parents," picked up a few Alien masks to try to lift the spirits of their son, Coleton, then 12, when he spent an excruciating Halloween night at the hospital. He was undergoing treatment for Ewing's Sarcoma, an especially cruel cancer that causes tumors to form on tissue and bone.

Coleton wasn't much in the mood for dress-up that night, but he thought he should play along for the sake of others. He wore his false face for the candy deliveries. But at the end of the night, when Danielle lifted the mask off her son's face, she found that it was all wet inside.

"He had been crying his eyes out the whole time," Danielle says, "hiding his tears from everyone."

Here's a thing you need to know about kids with cancer: They often wear masks – metaphorically, that is. Even when they feel down, they put on a brave face. They feel as if they should not inconvenience friends, family, and hospital staff with talk of their troubles.

"I tried to always keep a smile on and distract," Coleton tells me. "Because you're not just staying positive for yourself, it's for the people around you, too."

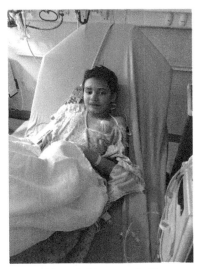

Coleton in his cancer battle.

In each of my three cancer battles, positivity has been a must. But positivity on the outside doesn't help the sorrow inside. Let me tell you, sometimes staying positive takes an emotional toll.

Kids like Coleton are given painful procedures to stay alive. That brings with it a complex set of emotions. And, too often, deep depression.

FACT: Childhood cancer survivors are 57 percent more likely to develop depression than kids without.
- JAMA Pediatrics peer-reviewed 2023 study.

"During chemo all those months, depression was huge," Coleton says. "I felt like I was trapped in my brain most of the time – outside of the real world. It was a dark place. You get used to being bald and falling asleep in car rides because you're so tired and can barely breathe from all the treatments. It got very grim, but I just kept pushing."

Depression comes with the reality that you're no longer living a normal life, at least compared to your healthier friends.

"I remember I picked Coleton up from a friend's house where it seemed like he was having a great time," Danielle recalls. "Then he got in the car and started bawling. He said, 'I just want to be normal.' "

Normal. There's a word that takes me back to a painful place in my own childhood.

I lost vision in my left eye in an accident with a pencil around 4 years old. After that, my eye would drift, leaving me incapable of looking people directly in the eyes. I remember in adolescence sitting in my room crying while I stared in the mirror.

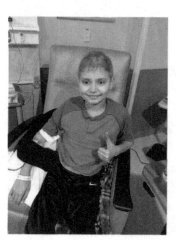

Coleton in his cancer battle.

The other kids would mock me mercilessly. I never wanted to tell a teacher or a coach because I didn't want to seem soft or have anyone feel sorry for me. Even though that feeling of not being normal cut me like a knife, I tried to never let my hurt show.

That was my mask.

And that's why my heart breaks for kids like Coleton who have their sense of normalcy stripped away. It's a hidden form of pain in a cancer battle that can be worse than many of the treatments they endure.

Not all, though.

"There was this one type of chemo called Doxorubicin that was nicknamed 'The Red Devil,' " Coleton tells me.

The Red Devil? Now we're talking real Halloween fright.

"It's because it would make your tears and sweat turn red from all the toxins," Coleton says. "You'd have mouth sores and couldn't eat solid food. It felt like your mouth had just gone through barbed wire.

"I remember one time on my birthday and my family made all this amazing food – steak, lobster. I couldn't eat any of it. That drug didn't allow me to do normal things with my family and it put me in a low place."

Doxorubicin, around since the 1960s, is a drug so intense that people who get treated with it are given lifetime maximums of use. Coleton faced the maximum of six treatments (due to his weight), meaning he can never legally ingest the brutal drug again.

"There were families we knew where their kids would be 15 and say, 'I don't want to do the chemo anymore' and they'd say okay, knowing the outcome (cancer leading to death) if they didn't," Danielle says. "We were going to drag him to (treatments) to save him if we had to."

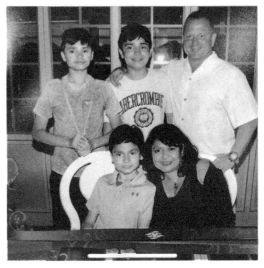

Coleton with his family.

Coleton turned to his drawings and art to help him cope. But things got even more grave.

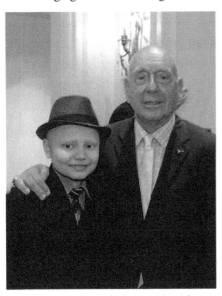

Dick and a young Coleton at the gala.

After a major surgery in December of 2018, Coleton had to re-learn how to walk, how to talk, even how to use his body for basic functioning. "It felt like I had to re-learn everything," he says.

Once again, that sense of normalcy was obliterated.

"The initial feeling after I was diagnosed was just emptiness," Coleton says. "Then it was just a long, arduous process. I thought the chemo would go through my body and all the chemicals would shrink the tumor, then it would be one quick surgery. That I'd be all done after that.

"I was so wrong."

Coleton's battle was grueling. Ewing's Sarcoma patients are given a combination of four chemos – two every other week for 14 weeks. He faced six rounds of chemotherapy in nine months. And then, midway through treatment, doctors removed 6 ½ inches of his right fibula. (He's still able to walk and run just fine without it.)

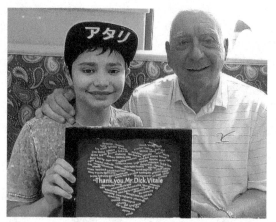
Coleton with a gift for Dickie V.

"It was never easy," Art says. "When the doctors would come in, he'd put his head under his sheets. But we had to keep pushing him. It was almost like being in the military."

Ryan Joseph is our photographer at the V Foundation who is actually in his own current battle with cancer. He is a friend of the Korney family and one day Ryan called to tell me about Coleton's diagnosis. He gave me Art's number, and I called right away.

"I was thinking, 'Why is Dick Vitale calling me?' " Art recalls. "You told me, 'We have a mutual friend, I heard your son just got diagnosed.' I said, 'Yeah, like seven minutes ago!' "

I told Art that I knew professional baseball players who had the same type of cancer and they got back on the field. I told him if Coleton needed better doctors or a better hospital, I'd make some calls from the network Lorraine and I have built over the years.

"I went from a state of oblivion to hope that our family could get through this," Art tells me. "It was like you *knew* you had to call at that exact time."

You're damn right I knew. Once I heard about Coleton's diagnosis, it was like the Bat Signal went up in the sky. All I could think about was the devastation that families go through after parents hear those four heartbreaking words: *Your child has cancer.*

The memory with Art has an even stronger meaning because of his own diagnosis with adenocarcinoma lung cancer – news that I sadly received during the publication phases of this book. The Korneys are among the many families who have multiple family members come down with cancer. *Unfair* doesn't even begin to describe their circumstances.

In Coleton's battle, the Korneys had several misdiagnoses at first, which is sadly quite common with Ewing's Sarcoma. Then a lump on his right calf grew from three centimeters to nine in mere weeks – before finally determining it was cancerous. Doctors had previously said it was lymph nodes and that treatment could wait. Boy, were they wrong.

> *I went from a state of oblivion to hope that our family could get through this. It was like you knew you had to call at that exact time.*
>
> *- Art Korney when Dick Vitale called him seven minutes after Coleton's cancer diagnosis.*

"I didn't trust many of the doctors after that," Danielle says. She is a force as a mother, let me tell you. Once she drove across the Sunshine Skyway Bridge to get her son his Neupogen shots when Hurricane Rita kept the manufacturer from being able to deliver them. She kept a journal on what the family went through and regularly posted on social media about cancer fighters.

Danielle wrote in a journal passage, after finding out Coleton had cancer: *Slammed against me like an ocean wave and I couldn't breathe. I gasped for air trying to understand what (the doctor) was saying but I couldn't hear past his first words. …I glanced over and my husband's face was flushed white in disbelief. Then he hugged Coleton while they both cried. Thank God he was there to comfort Coleton while I turned into Spock from Star Trek.*

"People would unfriend me and duck if they saw me at the grocery store," Danielle says. "For many people in our circle, it was like it hit too close to home when you see a kid going through cancer."

How sad is that? Not only is your family in the fight for your kid's life, but then you're stuck losing your sense of community. The Korneys did their best to replace neglectful friends with meaningful ones.

Danielle encouraged Coleton to be a mentor to Seth Ybarra, a fellow cancer patient who was just beginning his journey. The two would connect over treatments and play video games together virtually.

"You realize that you need people in your life going through the same or similar things," Danielle says. "I remember one time Coleton had come out of his surgery and he's like, 'Where's my phone? I need to text Seth to tell him it's not as bad as you think it'll be in your head.' "

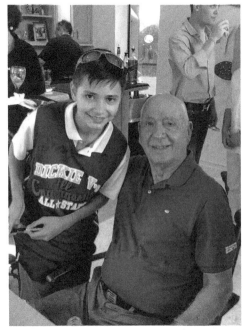

Dick and Coleton, in his All-Courageous Team jersey.

Coleton's mentoring of Seth came on the heels of his friend Corey LaFave mentoring him. Sadly, Corey did not make it in his own battle with Ewing's Sarcoma, but Coleton says he'll "always be grateful for that friendship."

"One day, I would like to start a program at hospitals that pairs up new chemo patients with mentors," Coleton wrote in his award-winning essay for the *Sarasota Herald-Tribune*.

Hey, Coleton has a point – and a purpose – with this mentoring thing. And he has so much to teach all of us. That's because Coleton's cancer story is as much about the aftermath as the actual battle. All that sadness he pushed down to spare others kept his pain hidden. And then it grew into full-blown depression.

He's hardly alone in this. A 2023 peer-reviewed study by *JAMA Pediatrics* showed that childhood cancer survivors are 57 percent more likely to develop depression than kids without.

"You don't just walk away from cancer," Danielle says. "It's not chicken pox. He's had all these bouts of depression and a lot of that stems from the fact that he's never going to be back to being him."

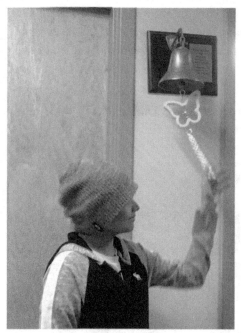

Coleton ringing the bell after his final cancer treatment.

Coleton rang the bell in May of 2018. He was, at last, cancer-free. Then, right as he was getting back into the swing of life, came the COVID-19 lockdown a year and a half later.

"I went from having cancer where I couldn't see any of my friends to not being able to see anyone because of the pandemic," Coleton says. "My high school experience was far from normal."

Like many his age, he struggled with the lack of connection to others. Here he was trying to get back to normal in the most abnormal of times.

"I was probably in the darkest place, but what really helped me was going to your galas," Coleton tells me. His first one was in 2018 and he says that gala and the mask-wearing 2020 gala (during the pandemic) were the most special. "That first gala brought me out of my shell because when I was done with chemo, that was the first big event I was at. At first, I was shocked because there were close to a thousand people there. The galas ended up being like the light at the end of the tunnel after being in isolation so long."

That warms my heart. Putting these cancer survivors on the same team can be beneficial in multiple ways, and Coleton tells me some of his All-Courageous teammates helped him big time.

"Some of the time we talk about cancer and our experiences, trying to help each other," he says of being with the other All-Courageous kids. "But most of the time we talk about living, the future."

> *The galas ended up being like the light at the end of the tunnel after being in isolation so long.*
>
> *- Coleton Korney on attending Dick Vitale's pediatric cancer galas.*

The future is a beautiful thing to behold for kids who, as Danielle puts it, "got so used to fearing tomorrow. Kids shouldn't have to worry like that. They deserve to live in a world where tomorrows are exciting, not exhausting."

Coleton's tomorrows are beginning to get brighter. He tells me about his latest trips to New York, touring the Big Apple for the first time, and Comic Con in nearby Tampa (the Korneys live near me in Lakewood Ranch). He revels in his new job as a barback at a local

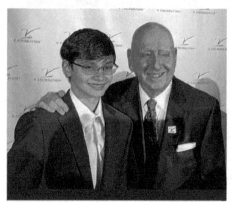

Coleton and Dick at his gala.

restaurant. He's still engaged with his own art and drawings. And he's studying art and business at State College of Florida full-time.

"Bits and pieces of happiness keep flowing in," Coleton says. "Living a normal life, doing normal things, changes your worldview."

He's out of isolation. The world is coming back to normal. He is, too.

"Since he's been around other people, more and more, his personality's exploded," Art says.

"He's always been able to wear his heart on his sleeve," Danielle says. "I'm glad cancer didn't take that away."

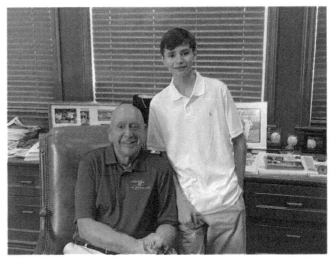

Coleton and Dick in his office.

Her son's personality has always been there, she says. It's just that cancer stunted it for a period of time. Now, more than five years cancer-free, Coleton's carefree personality is blossoming.

No masks needed.

To donate to the V Foundation, Dick Vitale Pediatric Cancer Research Fund, please scan this code.

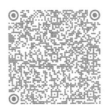

Chapter
Eleven
Discovering Your Inner Voice
with the Mikari Tarpley Family

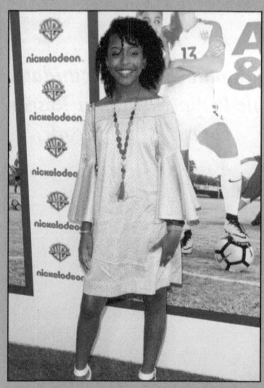

"For People of Color, our light is very small in the performing arts realm. I want to change that."

- Mikari Tarpley

Hakuna Matata.

It means "no worries," as Mikari Tarpley knows so well. She played young Nala in the national touring production of *The Lion King* when she was 11.

Then, just five years later, she was diagnosed with Hodgkin's lymphoma.

No child should have such worry as that.

Her diagnosis came on March 20 of 2020, barely a week after the national shutdown for the COVID-19 pandemic.

"It was literally two awful things happening at the same time," Mikari tells me of her micro and macro adversities hitting all at once.

The murder of George Floyd came two months later. It galvanized a national protest movement against police brutality – Black Lives Matter. Mikari ached to join in, but her illness left her immunocompromised, and the lymphoma treatments left her weakened. (Hers is a type of cancer where white blood cells grow out of control and cause swollen lymph nodes.)

That June, for her 16th birthday, she canceled her previously planned Sweet 16 party – and instead set out to raise $16,000 with a fundraiser dedicated to helping children with sickle cell blood disorders. This came a week before her final round of chemotherapy, mind you.

Mikari organized the fundraiser through the Aflac Cancer and Blood Disorder Center of Children's Healthcare of Atlanta. According to the Center for Disease Control, sickle cell disease affects one of every 365 African-American births, and the sickle cell trait (SCT) is present in one of every 13.

"When I was at the hospital for my treatment, there were maybe two brochures for sickle cell and like a hundred for all the cancers out there," Mikari says. "I

Dick with Mikari and her dad.

wanted to support my community – Black people who need it – and especially kids who don't understand what they're going through.

"I just wanted to do something in my capacity. I was able to start my own personal movement."

The fundraiser exceeded its goal and reached $20,000. My friends, Mikari is special. Instead of focusing only on her own cancer, she thought of others in her community.

FACT:
Sickle cell disease affects one of every 365 African-American births,
and the sickle cell gene is present in one of every 13.
- Center for Disease Control

This is what I've tried to do myself in the fight against pediatric cancer. We often ask ourselves when hit with some serious adversity: *How am I going to respond?* Well, as Mikari says, "You realize there's no benefit to staying in the wallowing emotions. You have to admit sometimes, like, 'Yeah, this sucks, I wish I didn't have to go through it,' but don't let that take away opportunities to laugh and find light in a dark time."

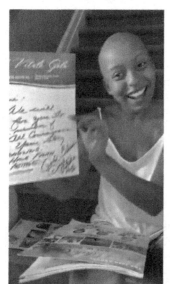

Mikari during her treatment with a letter from Dick.

Cancer didn't stand a chance against that mindset.

Still, she didn't have an easy go of it. Mikari came down with a fever during her first wave of chemotherapy, which was given to her on three consecutive days. Mikari counter-punched with a restructured plan that allowed her more rest between treatments.

"I knew I was in for a journey, but I just told myself it was something I could tell my kids about one day," she says.

The day-by-day of her cancer battle showed Mikari how to "lead with love" but she had to dig down deep and get gritty to attain that approach.

She writes in a scholarship she won for the National Children's Cancer Society: "Every week, I was nauseous because everything reminded me of the radioactive fluids coursing through my veins in the infusion room. My mouth reeked of a metallic taste every day. Some days my body hurt so much that I couldn't get out of bed. So yes, in many ways, I was broken. But chemo did not break me completely. The one thing that consistently got me through my five months of treatment was the small voice in my head saying, 'You were meant to fight this fight for a reason.' When I doubted whether I could be stronger than this disease, the voice would cry out, 'Fight it, conquer it, and live to tell your story.'"

Mikari's parents felt a natural urge to protect their daughter at first, but they quickly recognized they had raised a warrior poised to become battle tested. "She was quick standing up and fighting against it. We sort of just followed her lead," says her father, Michael. "Even at that age, she'd become a natural leader and that's probably what's allowed her to lead others to this day."

Mikari, 19 now, is in her second year at Howard University, in Washington, DC, where she is studying to get her Bachelors of Fine Arts degree in Musical Theater. It's fitting considering how she confides "the arts saved me" during her cancer bout and the pandemic.

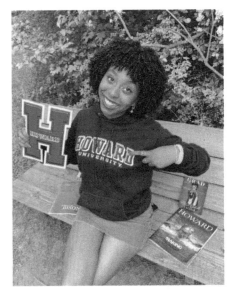

Mikari at Howard University.

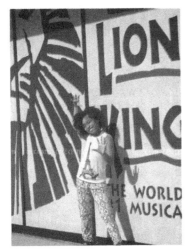

Mikari was in the Broadway tour of The Lion King.

She had a supporting role in the 2018 Warner Brothers film, *Alex & Me,* and she made an appearance in an episode of the Oprah Winfrey-produced *Queen Sugar*. And, of course, she was Young Nala in the Broadway tour of *The Lion King* that crossed North America in 2015-2016.

Mikari doesn't want to be a performer for the glitz and glamour. Instead, she says, it's all about inspiring others. Count me as one of those who is inspired big time by this special lady.

"Fighting cancer gave me this renewed perspective," she tells me. "I sort of realized, 'If I'm going to exist, I'm going to exist for a reason.' I needed to have more meaning. I want to make a mark and stand out so that I can empower other people in so many different ways. (The performing) arts can be powerful because it can move people. Stories through performance can help speak for those who can't speak for themselves. Especially for people of color, our light is very small in the performing arts realm. I want to change that."

Fighting cancer gave me this renewed perspective. I sort of realized, if I'm going to exist, I'm going to exist for a reason.

- Mikari Tarpley

I came to know Mikari in 2020 when she wrote me a beautiful letter that I still keep to this day. (A good friend of mine, former NFL fullback Rob Robertson, had suggested that she reach out to me.) Then I posted a video on social media reading her letter to all of my followers. I must have said "wow" a dozen times. That's how taken I was with her words.

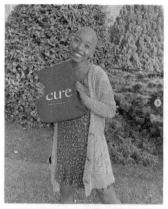

Mikari during her cancer battle.

"We didn't expect you to read the letter to the whole world," Mikari says, chuckling. "I could see how much you cared when you read it."

How could I not? Here is part of what she wrote:

"Upon learning (of the diagnosis), I had the same thought so many battling cancer do: *Am I going to make it? Am I going to die?*"

That thought is inevitable – trust me, I know – and debilitating, too. But for a teenage girl to have to ponder that?

"I know it's not smart to think like this," she wrote, "so I went about living life normally. …I try to cherish each day like it's a blessing. Because it's not granted. There is no saying you or me will wake up tomorrow, so you just have to enjoy every day."

She has wisdom beyond her years, absorbing life as a gift instead of a privilege. Take a look at this Instagram post she made while she was still battling cancer:

"I'm here and I'm alive. So to whoever is reading this, be thankful for where you are and what you have. Be thankful that you woke up this morning. Be thankful that even if you aren't where you want to be in life right now, you still have a life to live. There is too much hate and evil in this world to ignore the good and constant blessings in your life. Even if you don't see them, they're there."

Like so many in this book, every special kid has a set of parents who help shape them. Enter Michael and mother Tomaree, two All-Star parents from a musical standpoint. Michael is a jazz saxophonist. Tomaree is a recording artist who had a 2013 single that was top-10 on the UK Soul Chart.

"When she first got cancer, the news was overwhelming and knocked us off our feet," Michael says. "But there was no 'why me' or pity party much at all."

Tomaree recalls washing Mikari's hair and big globs of it coming out: "I kept saying, 'I'm not going to cry.' I was having a hard time keeping it together but this whole time, this chick is laughing and being funny. That really helped some of those moments become bearable – her ability to make light of things."

Because Mikari's chemo treatments coincided with the pandemic's early days, her parents could not see her together due to a hospital protocol of one visitor at a time. The need to stave off any viruses when she was immunocompromised remained at the forefront the whole time.

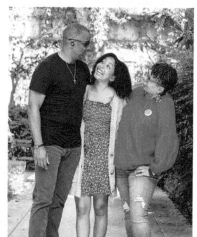

Mikari with her parents.

"That made it tough," Tomaree says. "But we had 100 nurses available to us and there was no traffic going into the hospital. And then because school was on hiatus, it allowed her to focus on her health 100 percent."

"Looking back at it now, Covid ended up making things easier in a way," Michael says. "It was almost like God saying, 'I'll take you through this and pave the way.' Even though she was going through cancer, there wasn't much outside of the actual (battle) that was stressing us out."

> *Cancer has taught me that I want to leave this world a better place.*
>
> *- Mikari Tarpley*

Mikari says she is almost grateful for her cancer ordeal in this respect: "Cancer has taught me that I want to leave this world a better place."

She has already done that for me. When I was fighting my vocal-cord cancer this past summer, Tomaree sent me the music video of a song by Syndee Winters, who played older Nala to Mikari's young Nala in that touring production of *The Lion King*. Mikari helped Syndee write the lyrics for "Warrior," a song about fighting cancer, and is featured on the track as well.

One line goes: "My voice is weak but my will is stronger." Damn, that hits home for me! Those lyrics helped me come to realize something about my battle with vocal-cord cancer: It isn't just a fight to regain my actual voice. It is also a fight not to let cancer silence my inner voice – my spirit, so to speak.

"I'll fight for my life. I'll fight for what's right," the song goes. "I'm a soldier. I'm stronger, a warrior."

One warrior to another, Mikari, thank you.

I've spent so much time being a coach in this fight against pediatric cancer that you need a little fine-tuning once you're playing the game, baby!

I know I've often thought of cancer as an opponent, a blasted nemesis that needs to be defeated. While the Tarpleys share that feeling, they also pointed out we can learn from our enemies.

Tomaree says: "You might go to school to take tests, but God gives us tests so we can learn a lesson."

That lesson, Mikari says: Her no-worries days are gone, but her true inner voice has been ignited.

"It's almost like a butterfly effect," she says. "Cancer is not something I'd wish on anyone. But I can tell anyone who does

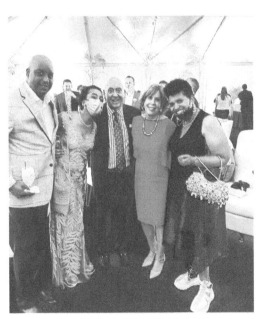

Michael, Mikari, Dick, Lorraine, and Tomaree at the gala.

93

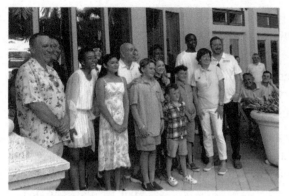

Mikari and All-Courageous Team members posing during the post-gala picnic at Dick's home.

go through it that, if you're fortunate to come out of it, you'll come out a better person for having fought it. In that way, I find myself almost grateful for what I've been through."

We've got a lot of troubles in this world, but with warriors like Mikari determined to make it better, I know we're going to be in good hands.

Hakuna Matata.

To donate to the V Foundation,
Dick Vitale Pediatric Cancer Research Fund,
please scan this code.

Chapter

Twelve

Unrelenting Faith

with the Josh Fisher Family

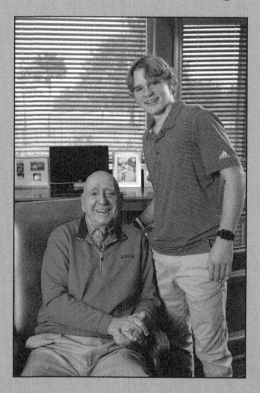

> *"Faith is the foundation for all of it. I just realize,*
> *looking back, that it was all in God's hands.*
> *He did everything with me on my journey."*
> *- Josh Fisher*

Patrick and Jessica Fisher prayed all night after their two-year-old son, Josh, was given a preliminary diagnosis of Acute Myeloid Leukemia, an aggressive type of cancer that can develop rapidly.

"We prayed more than we ever have before," Patrick tells me. "We said, 'God, make this somehow treatable or curable. We'll do our part, you do your part.' "

The next day, Josh's oncologist came in and said that the "strangest thing happened." Josh's cancer scans came back as lymphoblastic, drastically changing the diagnosis. Josh's odds of winning his fight against cancer improved from 30 percent to 85 percent overnight.

"The doctor said it's something that had never happened before," Patrick says. "He told us he ran the test three times just to be sure because they were so surprised by the change."

The Fishers prayed, and the way they see it, their prayers were answered.

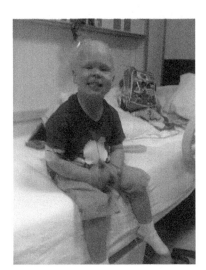

Josh during his cancer battle.

"We truly believe God heard our prayers and changed Joshua's cells overnight," Jessica says. "After we learned that, we were, like, 'We got this. Let's get through this with Josh and be the light to other people if we can.' We didn't go the route of, 'Why was Josh chosen to be different?' We were able to accept (the diagnosis) because we felt like we received a miracle and that it was going to be okay – in His hands."

The Fishers aren't the only family to try to make a deal with God. Lord knows that's a common theme for cancer-stricken families after hearing heartbreaking news. And I can't tell you how many parents have told me over the years they prayed for God to give them cancer so that it could be taken away from their kids.

I know about mistaken diagnoses all too well. When my original diagnosis of bile-duct cancer was changed to the more treatable lymphoma in 2021, it meant no surgeries and a clearer treatment plan, with less mindboggling decision-making. I remember celebrating the lesser diagnosis. It was like Christmas came early, baby!

You wouldn't think that someone would ever be celebrating any cancer diagnosis, but sometimes it's truly a matter of perspective. Those original diagnoses were not easy to accept for the Fishers or for me, let me tell you. But they made the updated ones a hell of a lot easier to accept.

Once I got to that point of acceptance in my first bout, in 2021, and then the second time around, in 2023, it allowed me to gain perspective and appreciate the little things in life – like my routine of going out to breakfast in the morning. Then there are the big things in life – like the daily miracles when my family members would drive me to treatments and support me, all with their own good health.

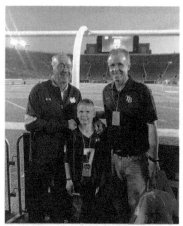

Dick with Josh, and his dad, Pat, at a Notre Dame game.

As I write this, I'm visiting my grandchildren at Notre Dame for a football game against Ohio State. (The Buckeyes snuck away with a last-second 17-14 win). Lorraine and I always try to take an annual trip to South Bend ever since both of our daughters played tennis for the Fighting Irish. We especially love going now that granddaughter Sydney and grandson Ryan are enrolled, too.

Fittingly, it brings me back to a time when I had Patrick and Josh Fisher join me for a Notre Dame football game against USC, back in 2017, right around the time that Josh finally rang the bell to be cancer-free at age 9.

"I remember you took my hat so you could blend in on the golf cart when we were on campus because everyone notices you," Josh reminds me.

Usually, I love people coming up to me when I'm on a college campus. But on that day, it was all about Josh, so it was better to go incognito. I remember throwing the football with Josh and he was having an absolute blast.

I didn't turn him into a Notre Dame fan that year, but Josh did eventually become an Ohio State fan when he became close pals with Urban Meyer, then the coach of the Buckeyes, through one of my galas years ago.

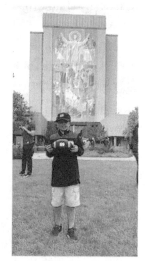

Josh at Notre Dame in front of "Touchdown Jesus."

"Urban was so nice to Josh and they got along so well," Patrick says. "Then I realized, we have a problem."

Both Patrick and Jessica are die-hard Michigan Wolverines fans. And, let me tell you, that Ohio State-Michigan rivalry was as heated then as it is now.

I love that Terri and Sherri and my grandchildren went to Notre Dame because not only is it one of the top schools in the country, it's also deeply rooted in the Catholic tradition. Every time I visit, I try to go to the Grotto of Our Lady of Lourdes, a rock cave built in 1896 that's used by visitors as a sacred space for prayer and meditation.

When I returned to the Grotto this past fall, it was after I had heard the preliminary news that doctors could not see any cancer around my vocal cords. But because the radiation did a number on my voice, they were waiting for it to clear up to determine if I was indeed cancer-free. So when I went to pray in the Grotto, I was grateful to God for helping me to get through my six grueling weeks of radiation treatment. But I was also praying for those words every cancer patient desires to hear from their doctor: *You're cancer-free.*

Praying has always been a big part of my life and, make no mistake, my faith is a huge part of who I am. It's not like I got cancer and then decided to get on my knees to the Man Upstairs. I haven't missed a Catholic Mass on Sunday for close to 30 years. Even when I'd be on a rigorous travel schedule in my heyday of calling college hoops games, Lorraine and I would find a Catholic church or chapel to attend or sometimes we'd even have a priest visit a hotel room for Communion. I like the structure and the routine of going to Mass, and that's mainly because I draw so much strength from my faith – as do so many families with their own faiths in their own cancer fights.

Both my parents were uneducated, but they had doctorates in love. …Now that I've had time to reflect since their passing, I understand better where they got those doctorate degrees from. They got their reservoir of love from their faith in Christ.

- Dick Vitale

I believe in my religion strongly and, at the same time, I respect the beliefs of others just as much. My religious beliefs were instilled in me by my parents, John and Mae. They were hard-working people who modeled strong faith despite challenging life circumstances. My Dad pressed coats in a factory during the day and worked as a mall security worker at night.

Both my parents were uneducated, but they had doctorates in love. They taught me never to believe in the word "can't" and to always treat people with respect so that you can receive respect in return. Now that I've had time to reflect since their passing, I understand better where they got those doctorate degrees from. They got their reservoir of love from their faith in Christ.

Growing up, I watched my mother walk to church every day, dragging her leg because of her condition following a stroke. She passed on her love for St. Anthony of Padua and St. Jude to me as a young boy, and that's a tradition I carry on to this day. Every morning, like her, I pray for the intercession of St. Anthony, patron saint of lost items, and St. Jude, patron saint of hopeless causes and desperate cases.

I keep a holy card of St. Jude in my pocket and have since I was young. It's even more vital to have it now. Because when you're a cancer patient, hopeless causes and desperate cases are exactly what you're messing with on a daily basis.

One of the only things I found myself asking others for during my cancer battle was prayers. Nonstop prayers. I saw from my parents just how transformative and restorative prayers can be. And I see it now in families like the Fishers.

At the end of the day, prayers are about trust in a higher power. Trust that He will uplift you through difficult and trying times.

FACT:

Acute Lymphoblastic Leukemia, Josh's official diagnosis, carried an 85 percent survival rate as compared to the more deadly 30 percent survival rate of Acute Myeloid Leukemia, the preliminary diagnosis that changed overnight.
- National Cancer Institute

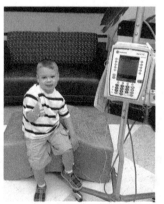
Josh during his cancer battle.

That trust was tested for Patrick and Jessica as they watched their son go through 1,200 doses of chemotherapy. You read that right: 1,200 doses over 3-½ years.

Patrick and Jessica are still haunted by the screams from all the side effects of his treatment – like when he'd have mini seizures or when his port had to be removed due to an infection. They were also tested when Justin and Charlie, their other boys, asked them – point blank – if Josh was going to die.

"We said to them back then: 'We're all going to die at some point. We don't know when God's going to take us,'" Jessica says.

As Jessica tells me this, Josh, now 15, interrupts her: "He'll take us to a better place than here on Earth when he does take us."

That's the mindset that Patrick and Jessica have instilled in Josh. He's got a spiritual perspective – embracing what heaven is all about – that outweighs fears of

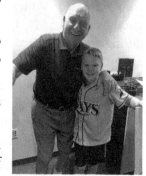
Josh and Dick hanging out.

dying in this life. I guess you have to face that fear when you grow up the way Josh did, with cancer looming.

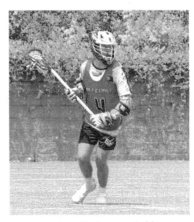

"We trusted God with everything," Jessica says. "That through God, as a family, we could overcome anything – even death."

"Being able to realize that truth gave us peace," Patrick adds.

Nowadays Josh is a successful lacrosse player in high school. (His parents were athletes, too. Jessica played college basketball and Pat was a ski racer). Josh is just as awe-inspiring now as he was during his fight with leukemia because his perspective in the game of life hasn't changed. It's a perspective that's reminded me during my own cancer fight that pain is temporary – and something you can overcome.

Josh on the lacrosse field.

"I was so young when I was going through cancer that it's hard to remember all of it, but looking back it was like my whole childhood was living in a hospital," Josh says. "One thing cancer taught me was how to maintain positivity as much as you can and not dwell in negativity. It's hard to maintain positivity and not become bitter. But it's best to just take things as they come and not think about something that hasn't happened yet."

Patrick and Jessica have worked as regional account managers for medical device companies, so they came into the cancer fight knowing medical terminology – and, crucially, who to call for care. They also recognize the blessing of keeping their family together, with Josh's brothers able to visit the hospital frequently during all those stays overnight.

Patrick and Jessica tell me they feel fortunate that they have stayed together. Sadly, that doesn't always happen in the case of couples with a kid in a cancer fight. That's why Patrick and Jessica founded their nonprofit for families in Central and West Florida called *BayStar Family Retreat*. It's meant to be a weekend of relaxation and much-needed respite for cancer-stricken families, where the emphasis is focused on repairing families on an emotional level. It emphasizes a Christian foundation of husband and wife and carries the slogan, "Be the Light in the Fight."

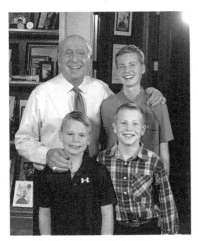

Dick with Josh, Cole Eicher, and Weston Hermann.

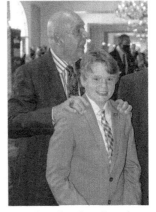

"While there are major large-scale strides being done on the medical side, the emotional and family support can take a backseat – with families struggling to find adequate small-

Dick with Josh at the gala.

scale help," Jessica says. "The premise of what we do is we pair a non-cancer family of volunteers with a cancer family. It's that other family's opportunity to give back and serve the family going through hardship. Those moments can really help towards keeping the cancer family intact."

Patrick says great organizations like Make-A-Wish center on cancer-stricken kids, but sometimes siblings in a family can feel neglected. The retreats aim to help families through those feelings.

"If you're a cancer family, everywhere you go, you're that cancer family," Patrick says. "But if you pair up with 10 other families, then you're no longer that family. It's an opportunity for Moms and Dads just to be themselves again and not in this constant cancer-fight mode."

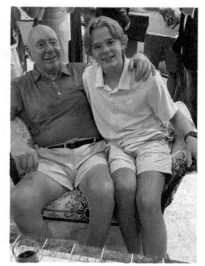

Dick and Josh at the gala picnic at the Vitale home.

> *Faith is the foundation for all of it. I just realize, looking back, that it was all in God's hands. He did everything with me on my journey.*
>
> *- Josh Fisher*

Patrick and Jessica tell me they've seen paired families stay in close contact over the years, forming deep friendships. The way the Fishers see it, they have a responsibility to pass on the light of God that was shone on them.

"Someone long ago created a pathway for Josh to have success in his treatments," Patrick says. "Now we just want to pay it forward so other kids don't have to suffer."

The Fishers, much like what my folks taught me, are paying it forward with love because they feel called on to do so.

"Faith is the foundation for all of it," Josh says. "I just realize, looking back, that it was all in God's hands. He did everything with me on my journey."

I'm not always the most avid reader of the Bible, I have to admit. But one verse stands out to me as we're talking about Josh. That verse – fittingly, Joshua 1:9 – reads: "Have I not commanded you? Be strong and courageous. Do not be afraid; do not be discouraged, for the Lord your God will be with you wherever you go."

The Fishers run their nonprofit, BayStar Family Retreat – serving families in Central and West Florida, with the aim of providing a relaxing weekend to cancer-stricken families. Their website is: baystarfamilyretreat.org

To donate to the V Foundation,
Dick Vitale Pediatric Cancer Research Fund,
please scan this code.

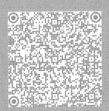

Chapter Thirteen

A Team of Superheroes

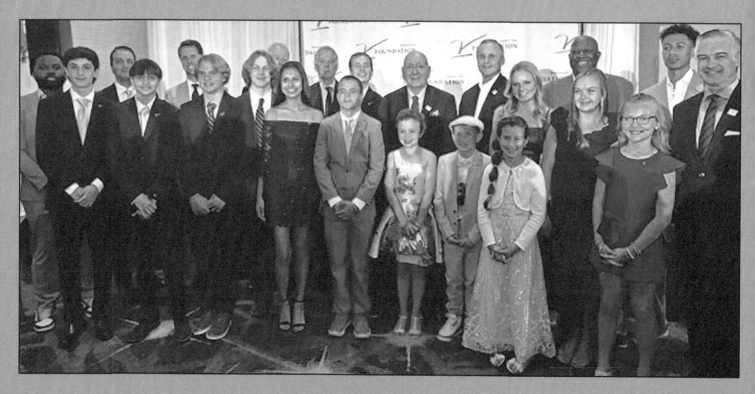

*"All of a sudden, I got swept out of my thoughts
of it being Dick Vitale versus cancer. It had become
the All-Courageous Team versus cancer."
- Dick Vitale*

I am a basketball broadcaster who always sees the game through the eyes of a coach. Hey, Coach K says so in the foreword to this book. And who am I to argue with the winningest coach in NCAA history?

The part I loved about being a coach with the University of Detroit and then the Detroit Pistons, in the 1970s, was the camaraderie that came from leading a team.

That's why I loved creating my own All-Courageous Team of superhero kids who fight cancer and showcase their abilities at my annual galas. I slipped right into the role I feel most comfortable in – as de facto coach.

But one thing that was never going to happen back in the days of disco, when I was coaching, was me miraculously shifting into a player-coach role. Not only was I too old, but I also could not run, or jump, or play defense. Even then, I had the body structure of linguine.

Yet on the All-Courageous Team, I'm the coach who gets to be a player. I will be one of the first to admit that there is an ugly irony to me getting cancer – all three times – considering I've made it my life's work carrying on Jimmy V's legacy in the fight to slay pediatric cancer.

Then again, maybe it's not so ironic in the big scheme of things. I don't exactly look at my own battles as blessings – far from it – but I'm not going to look at my cancers like they're a curse, either.

Look, I wouldn't wish cancer on anyone, but as I've opened my heart to kids going through these unfair battles, I can see how getting cancer in my 80s allows me to see the fight from their perspectives a little better.

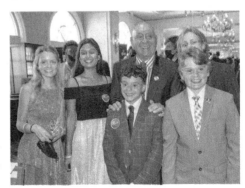

Dickie V with his All-Courageous Team kids.

These superhero kids display more courage than Superman and Spiderman put together, let me tell you. Our courageous kids have powers far beyond flying, X-ray vision or web-slinging. We're talking about the ability to persevere and show resiliency through endless chemo and radiation treatments when their friends are out playing sports carefree. We're talking about establishing a mental attitude that helps them overcome negative thoughts and hyper-focus on what's positive. And, of course, we're talking about my four Ds: Desire, Dedication, Determination, and Discipline of body and mind.

On the note of dedication, I will be the first to say: No winning coach recruits and guides winning team members without top-of-the-line supporting coaches. When it comes to my annual galas, the Olympic Games of my fight against pediatric cancer, there are no better bench partners than Mary Kenealy and Janet Allen of Mary Kenealy Events. For nearly two decades, my galas have been held in Sarasota as elite fundraisers because of the invaluable efforts of these two fabulous ladies. There would be no gala every year without this dynamic duo, and the All-Courageous Team families rave about their mastery at our events.

You've already had a chance to meet a handful of my active All-Courageous Team members in the prior pages, but like every winning program, there are foundational members and teams that help lay the groundwork for those who come after them. Even Coach K will tell you that his 1986 national-runner up team of Johnny Dawkins, Tommy Amaker, and Jay Bilas helped set the stage for those back-to-back championships that followed in the 1990s. Without the '86 squad, there is no Christian Laettner or Bobby Hurley the way we know them.

Similarly, the All-Courageous Team has some founding members and key players who continue to make this team super-heroic. So, allow me to introduce you to some of the real-life superheroes who helped shape my All-Courageous Team.

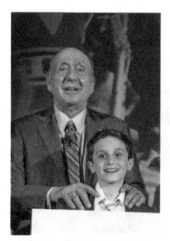

Jared with Dick at his gala.

Jared Rascio

Little did Jared know when I asked him to be on my team that the experience would be similar to what's in the comic books and superhero movies that he loves.

"When you go through cancer, you become part of this club with other cancer survivors, but it's not exactly a club you want to be in," Jared tells me. "With the All-Courageous Team, everyone has different backgrounds. They come from different parts of the country. And they've been through different types of cancer battles. So, when it's set up more like a team, you can see each member has their own unique abilities."

When Jared first went up on the stage at my annual gala, in 2015, as a member of the All-Courageous Team, the audience roared its approval

> *It feels like we're the Avengers. We're a group of kids brought together as representatives to fight for a common cause for good.*
>
> *- Jared Rascio*

with a standing ovation. He said it felt almost like he had been transported to another dimension.

"It feels like we're the Avengers," Jared says. "We're a group of kids brought together as representatives to fight for a common cause for good."

See? These kids really are superheroes and deserve to be treated as such. No one can convince me otherwise, baby.

What Jared feels is exactly why the All-Courageous Team was formed. As Lorraine and I started to know some of the mainstay kids better through our galas, I thought, "Why don't we form an actual team and pay tribute to all of the young people around the world who have had to deal with such a battle?" The message to cancer-stricken families around the world was simply this: If our team of youngsters can battle and beat cancer together, you can too.

The kids on my team all have these superpowers, but they don't acquire them without fighting a costly battle. Whereas Captain America was injected with a "super-soldier" serum, Jared was injected with methotrexate, a type of chemo drug to treat his leukemia.

"This was a drug that was bright, fluorescent green," says Jared's mother, Susan Lipton-Rascio. "It literally looked like something that came out of a superheroes' lab. It was practically glowing in the dark and hardly something you'd think could go inside a kid's body."

Susan is my agent with the Montag Group. I remember at a pediatric cancer event during the 2014 Final Four in Dallas, I was talking to her about how blessed we were to have healthy children and grandchildren. We talked about how unfair it was for parents to have to go through such a nightmare with their kids fighting this dreaded disease.

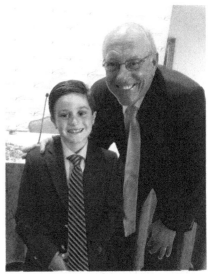

Jared with Jim Boeheim.

"Then that nightmare became real for us," Susan says.

Just a couple of weeks after that day in Dallas, Jared was diagnosed with Acute Lymphoblastic Leukemia. Before you knew it, Jared was starting up what doctors call the Induction Phase with four weeks of steroids and chemo meant to blast the leukemia out of his body. It's heartbreaking to me that families can be going about their lives normally in one instant and then have their worlds turned upside down the next.

"We were doing all these tests and I was in a state of denial," Susan says. "He was having what we'd call 'pain-ups' when he'd wake up in the middle of the night in excruciating pain. We later found out that was the leukemia in his bones trying to push its way out."

Jared went on to endure a 2 ½-year treatment of chemotherapy to negate any chance of the leukemia returning. I've watched the youngster, now 16, become someone I'm so proud to have in my life.

"I remember the child life specialist brought in these sock puppets," Jared tells me. "One sock was a white blood cell and it was acting like a police officer. The other sock was the cancer and it was the bad guy. When the puppets explained to me that I had cancer, I put my hands up to my cheeks like Macaulay Culkin in *Home Alone* and said "I caught cancer?" I then knew I had cancer but just didn't know exactly what it was."

Those cancer-fighting years, from ages 6 to 8, evaporated a normal childhood. We've talked about it throughout this book – this idea of how normalcy is ripped away from these kids. That's despite all the solid-gold attempts by family and hospital staffers to adjust that reality. What we see on the other side of that abnormal life experience are kids like Jared who perhaps return to normal activities for kids their age. But they're forever changed.

And the way I see it, they're forever superheroes.

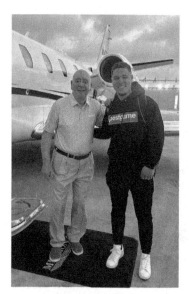

Jake posing with Dick in recent years.

Jake Taraska

Jake is a true veteran of the All-Courageous Team, someone who was there from the very beginning and turned into a team leader – the Batman or Ironman, if you will. Jake was diagnosed with neuroblastoma at 18 months old and his parents were told by doctors he likely wouldn't be able to walk or talk due to the severe side effects of the adult-sized treatments.

Turns out the doctors were wrong.

Jake went on to play college baseball at Keiser University in West Palm Beach as a relief pitcher despite having balance issues that plagued him intermittently throughout his childhood. He also worked through a stutter via many years of speech therapy.

"When I was little, growing up, my twin sister used to speak for me," Jake tells me. "She probably spoke for me most of the time up until I was 13 years old. I was scared of embarrassing myself."

Jake's superpower is truly evidenced in his then-to-now transformation. When you look at how he was, how he was forecast to be, and then the fact that he instead became someone he chose to be – or, better put, fought to be – that's supernatural in my book. Seriously awesome, baby.

He went on to create his own fundraiser, the *Jake Taraska Foundation*, in high school with the aim of helping cancer-affected kids on a micro level by raising funds for them to buy things like video games.

Nowadays he's the vice president of operations at Postgame, a company designed to help college athletes earn from their name, image and likeness. Talk about a company for the modern-day student-athlete.

His mother, Alli, says Jake's always had an enhanced work ethic in his DNA, perhaps because in many ways he had to do that throughout his life from the earliest stage.

"Jake always had to work double-time to measure up," she says. "He'd get to the (baseball) park early because as a pitcher the mound was elevated and he wanted to get his balance right before pitching in the game. He worked three times as hard and used his passion to become a great player. A lot of athletes have talent. Jake's talent was he'd work harder than anyone."

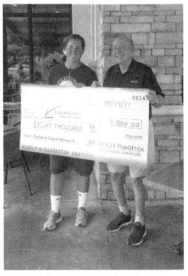

Jake presents Dick with a donation check to the V Foundation.

Few have been to more galas than Jake. He was at one of the first galas in 2009 and has only missed one since. (I still give him a hard time about missing it.) He was 10 at his first gala and kept on coming back, far removed from his cancer battle. Now, at 25, he's shifted into more of an honorary team member. Let's call him a player-coach.

I think you realized really early on that you had to kind of back up what you were preaching about these kids going through pediatric cancer. The All-Courageous Team is really the face of what you're trying to do. We've become the backbone to your fight against pediatric cancer.

- Jake Taraska to Dick Vitale

"I think you realized really early on that you had to kind of back up what you were preaching about these kids going through pediatric cancer," Jake tells me. "The All-Courageous Team is really the face of what you're trying to do. We've become the backbone to your fight against pediatric cancer."

I couldn't have said it better myself, Jake.

Tatum Parker

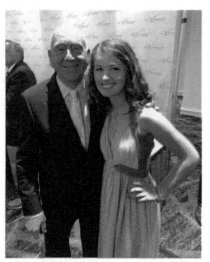

Tatum with Dick at an event.

Tatum is a two-time cancer survivor who is as tough as they come. She was diagnosed with Ewing's Sarcoma a couple weeks before her sixth birthday. She was in remission for 18 months, then cancer came back, this time in her right lung.

She became cancer free, for good, in 2009, but like many of the All-Courageous kids has suffered unfair side effects. She had to have her right hip replaced because of all the wear-and-tear from surgeries, and she has a metal part of her leg that strains on her when she walks.

Cancer didn't mess with Tatum's singing voice, though. She's an electrifying country singer and, oh my, can she belt the national anthem. She's a native of Indianapolis who was singing at Indiana Pacers and Notre Dame games when she was 12.

I came to know Tatum through Brad Stevens when he was coaching Butler University to back-to-back national runner-up finishes in 2010 and 2011.

What impressed me the most about Tatum was her drive to embolden others. She started her own nonprofit, the *Tatum Parker Project*, that's still working wonders to this day. The organization distributes backpacks – "Tatum's Bags of Fun" – that are filled with activities, games and toys for every child who is diagnosed with cancer in Indiana. Let me say that again – every single child diagnosed in the state of Indiana. That is absolutely Awesome, baby, with a Capital A.

> *It's a role reversal. You were always there for us to wish us well when we had big things going on with treatment. It's our turn to give back a little bit with the inspiration you gave us.*
>
> *- Tatum Parker to Dick Vitale*

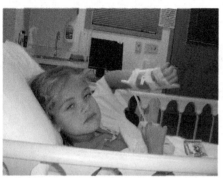

Tatum during her cancer battle.

"When I was first diagnosed, I received a bag of fun things," Tatum says. "It made me really feel loved and appreciated, like somebody's out there thinking about you and cares to see you through."

Tatum's one of the first kids to remind me how important it is to take life's obstacles and turn them into opportunities. And you better believe I tried to do that in my three bouts with cancer.

"I learned back then that you can't take anything for granted and you're never promised the next day," she says. "That perspective isn't something kids usually have to think about but I gained that perspective at six years old."

Now 23 and a fresh graduate of Indiana University in Bloomington, Tatum says it's easy to forget about the life lessons she once learned from her cancer battles.

"If I were to go back into a time machine, I could probably learn a thing or two from my younger self," Tatum says. "In a way, I was much more positive then and look what I was going through. It just goes to show that when you're not going through something as awful as a cancer battle, you can more easily lose sight of what's really important."

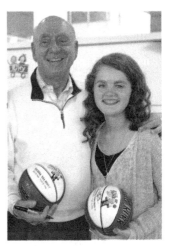

Tatum and Dick.

Nowadays, Tatum is student-teaching at her old school, Spring Mill Elementary, in Indianapolis. "I've always wanted to work with kids," she says. It figures. She's going to be teaching first grade, and her kids will be the same age she was when she was diagnosed with cancer.

"I'll get to heal my inner child," she says.

And true to her form, help others along the way.

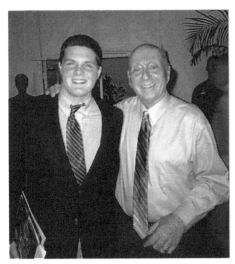

Kyle with Dick at his gala.

Kyle Peters

Kyle was 10 when he was diagnosed with brain cancer. He's a pure Prime Time Player and a huge part of the success of the galas over the years, let me tell you. He'll be forever tied to the legacy of what the All-Courageous Team is all about.

"I'm eternally grateful for being on the best team I could ever be on," he says.

Kyle had the same form of brain cancer that little Payton Wright died of a few short years before Kyle began his treatment that entailed extensive chemotherapy and radiation of his entire brain.

Kyle's triumphant survival and recovery from cancer felt so deeply full-circle for Lorraine and me because the more child-focused treatments that were unavailable when Payton was diagnosed were better equipped for Kyle's treatment. In large part thanks to the grant we started in Payton's name, Kyle says "more efficient and cleaner therapies were developed, and this resulted in a quicker, smoother recovery process for me."

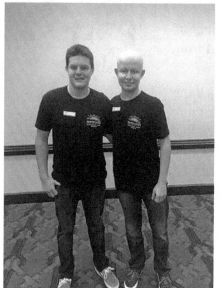

A younger Kyle with Tony Colton.

Kyle was also close friends with Tony Colton. In fact, when Kyle got cancer, it was Tony who shaved his head to show his support.

"His loss hurts to this day and has contributed to some of the survivor's guilt feelings I've had to work through," Kyle tells me. "When you go up there on the stage for the gala, you realize that not everyone has Stage 2 and will survive. Some have Stage 4 and unfortunately don't make it."

Kyle brings up a key point about losing team members. Because that's a reality we face on our team, a reality regular sports teams don't usually have to face. On our team, no one's graduating, transferring, or getting traded. Sadly, they lose their lives. That truth is what inspires me to wake up the day after we've raised $12 million from a gala and push even harder for the next year. The way I see this, it's tough to take a day off as coach of this team.

> *When you go up there on the stage for the gala, you realize that not everyone has Stage 2 and will survive. Some have Stage 4 and unfortunately don't make it."*
>
> *- Kyle Peters*

The harsh reality can also pave the way for grounded perspective. "Tony's loss has really helped me look at my life now as a second chance," Kyle says. "I have inspiration to do what I really want to do."

Kyle's been cancer-free since 2011 and is now the coordinator of Florida operations for the Pittsburgh Pirates. His mom, Jenn, says he's basically 24-going-on-40 because of what he's had to face in his life.

"Looking back on my experience with the galas as a kid," Kyle says. "I'm just so grateful because the celebrities and everything that came with them took my mind off of only being a cancer survivor as a kid and offered me this turning point to become more – as sort of a cancer spokesperson who can make a difference."

It's unfortunate that kids like Kyle aren't given a choice as to whether they want to take on the superhero mantle. It's hard business fighting for others after you've fought for yourself in ways no 10-year-old should ever have to. When I try to think about what the gala stage represents, Kyle points out it provided him doses of "refuge" after a storm. Because even after the battle's over, your world is still spinning.

I hadn't really processed Kyle's point that being up there in front of hundreds of people can offer respite. But it makes sense, considering the galas are built to help these kids feel accomplished and appreciated – like a soldier coming home from war.

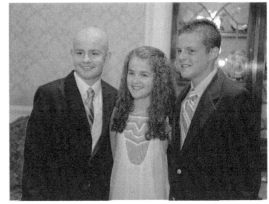

Tony, Tatum, and Kyle.

A Payback of Superhero Proportion

All this brings me to a moment that will stay locked in my heart forever. In the middle of my radiation treatment to address my vocal-cord cancer this past summer, I was truly down, feeling the side effects that included sore throat and difficulty swallowing. I was riddled with anxiety about whether I'd be able to use my voice again.

Just then, in my dark night of the soul, Lorraine tells me she has a video to show me from "my team." I didn't have to ask which team. I knew it was the All-Courageous kids.

The love and support that came pouring out of the video was tremendous and an emotional resuscitator when I needed it most.

Little Harper Harrell, an inspiring 10-year-old girl who battled Acute Lymphoblastic Leukemia and joined the team last year, blew kisses of support and told me: "I just wanted to say we all know you're so brave and we know you're even more brave when you have to go through something like this. You're acing it."

Jayden Spencer, an 18-year-old newbie to the team who battled Non-Hodgkins Lymphoma in 2022, told me: "Just know that your All-Courageous Team is behind you every step of the way. You'll get through this. Always remember: the tougher the battle, the stronger the person."

Sydney Hassenbein, 16 now after a bout with cancer that started at age 4, told me: "We know you can beat this. You're so inspirational to us all. And we need you to get through this."

Kinsley Peacock, a 10-year-old girl who had her right eye removed from a retinal tumor at age 5, told me: "We're thinking about you, we're praying for you, and you've got this. You're super strong." Kinsley has raised over $500,000 for her non-profit, *Kinsley's Cookie Cart*, and tells me she "loves being part of such a special team of warriors."

Everyone from this book made an appearance in the video, including Jared, who filmed his segment at one of my favorite places from my broadcasting career – on a college tour at Duke University. "I know you'll be back at Cameron Indoor Stadium soon enough," he said. "We're all praying for you and we love you."

Man, oh man. The whole team was there for me. Exactly when I needed them most. As we watched, Lorraine and I were brought to a waterfall of tears.

I mean, talk about strength in numbers. I had team members reach out to me separately during my first battles in 2021 and 2022, and their support always meant the world to me. But seeing all the kids have my back the way they did during my 2023 bout, well, it was something special, let me tell you.

> *All of a sudden, I got swept out of my thoughts of it being Dick Vitale versus cancer. It had become the All-Courageous Team versus cancer.*
>
> *- Dick Vitale*

Think of this: When 20-plus team members – kids I've dedicated my life to – tell you, "We're all here fighting with you," it resonates in such a profound way. Because you truly need that kind of support to win a battle like this. All of a sudden, I got swept out of my thoughts of it being Dick Vitale versus cancer. It had become the All-Courageous Team versus cancer.

"We weren't about to let you fight this alone," Jake tells me. Leave it to the veteran player-coach to offer me that.

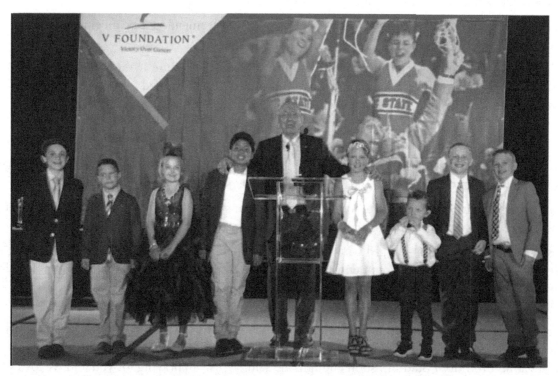

Dick and the All-Courageous Team at the gala.

It floors me to know how this team of cancer battlers at different times in their lives has been able to flourish for nearly two decades now.

"I just remember you always wanted to know more about my story and made it feel like we were the only two people in the room at your big event," says former team member Lindsey Rose Belcher. She's 22 now and get this: She's a pediatric oncology registered nurse at the same hospital – All Children's Hospital in St. Petersburg, Florida – that she was a cancer patient at when she was 7 to 10 years old. Talk about full circle, baby. "Being a nurse now, I work with the most inspiring kids in the world and every time one of them rings the bell, my 7-year-old heart lights up."

After my radiation treatments concluded this past fall, Dr. Matt Biagioli told me that the reason things went so well with my treatments was because of doing the little things like sleeping right, eating right, and maintaining a positive attitude. There's no way I could've done all those things without my All-Courageous Team behind me. No way.

I also had team members provide me small gifts and get-well cards that served as much-needed pick-me-ups.

One that stands out to me is from Joel McConkey, a 14-year-old youngster who passed out small inspirational cards at my 2023 gala. They were built to uplift people from his own 2020-21 battle with osteosarcoma, a rare but aggressive form of bone cancer that mostly affects children in their legs and arms. His testimony on the "Fight Like Joel" cards reference the bible verse, Job 23:10. The verse is fitting and inspirational. It centers on Job, who was obedient to God and trusted Him that he'll come out of the furnace of affliction as pure gold.

Man, can I relate to Job. I went into the furnace of radiation for six straight weeks when I would wear a giant protective layer over my face, neck, and chest. Coming out of the radiation furnace made me feel like pure gold at times, let me tell you. Because here I am at 84 seeing through a lens of purpose.

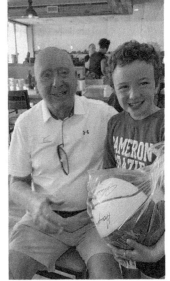

Another touching gift came from little Harper, who sent me a heartwarming note and a "Brave Like Harper" T-shirt before a pivotal surgery last July.

"You always put us in front of your own battles," she tells me. "You're such an enthusiastic man and we love you so much. I have people come up and tell me I'm their hero a lot, but I don't always feel like one. One time you tweeted that I was your hero, though, and I was like, *that* makes me feel like a hero because you're one yourself!"

That all brings me back to this notion of superheroes. I always thought the one major superpower that defines me was my voice. But I'm realizing

Harper Harrell and Dick.

through my All-Courageous Team members that when you're silenced, your voice can be heard in different ways.

Emily Ayers, 15, taught me this. When she was unable to speak fully due to side effects from her battle with Acute Myeloid Leukemia, she channeled her adversity by taking up ventriloquy with puppets. She got used to making sounds of characters without fully speaking and then later volunteered her time with this

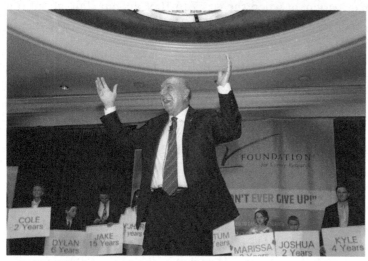

skill to younger kids battling cancer. She also has her own organization, *Emstrong Foundation*, which is centered on giving back to the organizations that helped her on her cancer journey, including the V Foundation.

"What goes around comes around," she tells me. "You get to pay it back."

People who know me well know that if there's a microphone in the room, I'm going for it. I love to speak. What can I say? Much of that is because I like to fight for others through my voice. Emily tells me that sometimes you have to let others speak for you – and in turn fight for you – too.

Dick celebrates cancer survivors on his All-Courageous Team at the gala.

"If you think about it, your whole team survived in a way because of how you helped them," she says. "Now it's the least we can do to help you. You encouraged us. Now we get to encourage you."

Pass the tissue, please.

Tatum echoes a similar sentiment to Emily's: "It's a role reversal. You were always there for us to wish us well when we had big things going on with treatment. It's our turn to give back a little bit with the inspiration you gave us."

Could a coach ask for a better team of superheroes?

To donate to the V Foundation,
Dick Vitale Pediatric Cancer Research Fund,
please scan this code.

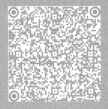

Chapter Fourteen
Hope as Lifeblood
with the Austin Schroeder & N'Jhari Jackson Families

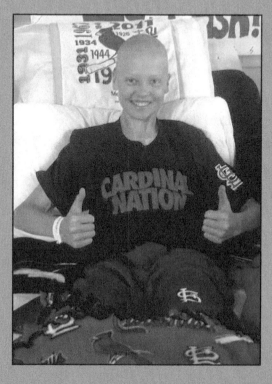

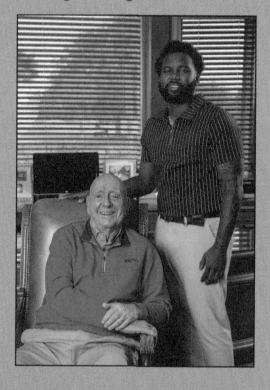

A man walks along a beach and sees a boy throwing something into the water. As he approaches, he sees hundreds of starfish lining the beach, washed in from the tide. The boy is throwing the starfish back into the water, one by one. "Why bother?" the man asks. "It's pointless. There are too many starfish to help them all." The boy flings another starfish deep into the water and says, "It mattered to that one."

My friends, so many times I feel like the starfish-throwing boy. And to me the man in the story can feel like the masses who won't listen when I plead for dollars to give these kids better treatments and life-saving research. The argument goes: We cannot invest funds into kids when their numbers don't compare to the quantity of cancer-stricken adults.

Look, cancer is a vicious disease. I get that it affects all of us and does not discriminate in age. (At 84, I can surely attest to that.) But this argument is backwards. It focuses on the macro scale of the issue – the sheer number of adults with a pressing need for treatments and, of course, an ultimate cure – versus zeroing in on the micro scale of the kids who need specified treatments just as much.

These kids are all starfish. It absolutely matters to the one. And let me tell you, when you invest in the one – particularly when it comes to these brave kids – you're also investing in the future to end this dreaded disease.

Here is why investing in the one is the right way to go – the only way, really: The kids who inspire us can then spread further inspiration out into the world, and that way we can experience a domino effect, baby!

I'm going to take you through the cancer experiences of two families. One of them lost their son. One still has theirs. Both stories showcase how providing a little bit of hope can work as an antidote to the devastation with which cancer so often poisons us in its aftermath. And – boy, oh boy – do both of these young men remind me of that boy saving the starfish.

We talked in the last chapter about superheroes. Now I want to tell you about a boy nicknamed "Flash" because he was the fastest kid on his football, basketball, and baseball teams. Austin Schroeder was his real name, and he and I became very close during his battle with cancer – one of the most horrendous encounters I have ever witnessed.

Iowa men's basketball coach Fran McCaffery is the one who called to tell me about Austin's story. Around the same time, Fran's son

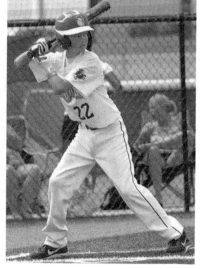

Austin at bat.

Patrick was fighting thyroid cancer. Patrick and Austin were close friends in the Iowa City area, both bare-knuckling cancer at the same time. Austin was diagnosed just a month after Patrick.

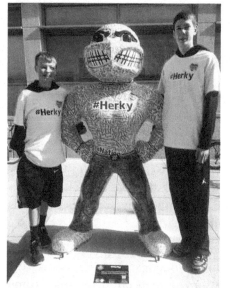

Austin with Patrick McCaffery in Iowa.

"Our families are connected in a way that is different than anything else," Fran tells me. "Our sons battled together and it's a bond we're grateful for because Patrick didn't have to go through it alone."

Fran was in the hospital with Austin and his family during our first phone call. "He was in so much pain and the family had just gotten devastating news," Fran recalls. "You called and all the sudden he was laughing and almost forgot about all his suffering – if only for a moment."

That wasn't a one-off phone call. I wasn't about to be a one-hit wonder to Austin, trust me.

We kept talking and getting to know one another. At one point, I gave him a shoutout during one of the games I was calling and eventually launched two grants in his name. It's my true calling to try to provide some form of hope for kids like Austin. One starfish always matters; you'll see why in a moment.

"Sometimes, the greatest gift you can give someone is hope," says Stacy Schroeder, Austin's mother. "Because hope is contagious once you have it. When Austin knew you were in his court, that you'd battle with him, it gave him what he needed in his battle."

> *Sometimes, the greatest gift you can give someone is hope. Because hope is contagious once you have it.*
>
> *- Stacy Schroeder*

"If you could've seen the look on his face when you called," says Craig Schroeder, Austin's father. "His face lit up like you wouldn't believe. He loved college basketball. You told him, 'Now you have my number and you can call anytime.' As a parent, we can't give our son that kind of support, a special gift like that. You let him know not to give up, that Dick Vitale is there with him."

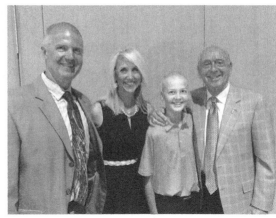

Dick with Austin and his parents.

Let me tell you, the feeling was mutual. I could tell when I was talking to "Flash" I was talking to someone with a unique ability to take on cancer, a kid who had the heart of a champion. Craig and Stacy have told me about how hard he battled.

When he was 14, after his initial diagnosis of T-cell Lymphoma, Austin was asked about what he could control. His point-blank reply: "My attitude and my effort." At a time when most people are in shock and defeat, Flash was lacing up his cleats for the biggest race of his life.

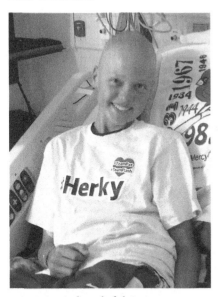

Austin bravely fighting cancer.

"That was who he was in a nutshell," Craig says. "His maturity level at such a young age was so beyond his years."

Craig, who was Austin's coach in baseball, came up with a motto of "win the day" long before the cancer diagnosis. It's got three components: Attitude. Effort. Shake N' Bake. (That last one means keep it light.)

"'Win the day' is not just about giving your best effort in sports but in all aspects of life," Craig says. "I would tell the kids, 'I want you to dive for the ball and give it your best. If you don't make a play, I just care that you go for it and give it your best.' It was about not being afraid to fail so you would not be afraid to succeed."

That mindset later translated into this: Austin not being afraid to die so that he wouldn't be afraid to live.

"At one point, towards the end, Stacy and I were wondering how much cancer had taken over his mind," Craig recalls. "I said to him, 'Hey, do you know why we had family visit you this weekend?' He said, 'Yeah, I could die any day now.' I asked him, 'Are you scared?' He said, 'I think it stinks because I don't want to die. But if this is what God wants me to do, I'll be watching over all of you every single

> *I asked him, 'Are you scared?'*
> *He said, 'I think it stinks*
> *because I don't want to die. But*
> *if this is what God wants me*
> *to do, I'll be watching over all*
> *of you every single day.' ...He*
> *understood this greater calling.*
>
> *- Craig Schroeder*

day.' It was awesome for us to hear that, because we sensed that he wasn't afraid. He understood this greater calling."

You don't get to that point of acceptance in your life purpose, as a gosh-darn 14-year-old kid, unless you focus on the micro picture – winning every day – instead of over-focusing on the macro picture that often turned out to be diagnoses or setbacks telling him dire news.

Remember, as my friend Stuart Scott put it, winning against cancer doesn't mean you stay alive. It's *how* you live. Austin epitomizes living every day like it's the last, and you better believe I took the Flash psyche with me in my own battles with cancer.

Austin's mindset was almost uncanny with how he channeled positive thinking amidst an ongoing storm of bad news. He used to say regularly, "Things could always be worse." The whole time, with setback after setback, he focused on winning one day at a time.

After the first 30 days of standard chemotherapy, early on during his journey, doctors told the Schroeders that the treatment wasn't working. They said the cancer had spread to his chest. He then signed up for a more rigorous 28-day regimen. After the first week of that, it began to show signs of working. But after the second week, because the treatments were mainly fit for adults, Austin had a negative reaction to where he couldn't speak. Basically, the chemo drug was too strong and proved it could be deadly to him.

Shortly thereafter, doctors told the Schroeders the cancer had been contained in his stomach, chest, and groin, but they still needed to address a cancerous spot on his knee. They opted for a bone-marrow transplant to address that. Then Austin got to play in a baseball tournament and celebrate his 15th birthday. Alas, this respite was not to last. Austin had a seizure that brought him back to the hospital and it was bad news again. This time the cancer had blown back up in his stomach, chest, and now in his bone marrow to where it was in the CNS fluid around his brain.

Eventually it got to a point where there were no treatments left. Then Austin was given the so-called Train of Life speech.

"They tell you, 'We all get off the train, but now God is asking you to get off the train earlier than everyone else,'" Craig recalls. "We were floored by his response. He said, 'Thank you.' Every single time he had a chance to see anyone working in the hospital, he said, 'Thank you.' Because he knew they were doing all they could to keep him alive."

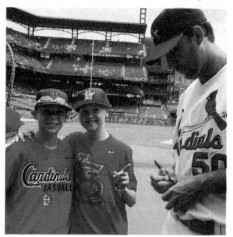

Austin on the field before
a St. Louis Cardinals game.

122

After being sent home on Hospice Care, Austin went back to the hospital one last time to sign a beam for the newly built University of Iowa Stead Family Children's Hospital. That's when Austin heard a mother crying in agony after heartbreaking news about her child: "Why is this happening to my baby?"

Craig distinctly recalls the moment: "He looked at us and said, 'This isn't fair. These other kids and parents don't know how to fight this. I need to beat cancer so I can come back to the hospital and show them what never giving up, finding the positives, and winning the day is about.' "

Austin, throughout his battle, always chose *how* to define what a win was. And now his wins are living on through his legacy.

"I just hope that if I go through something myself like that, I can handle it as well as he did," Craig says. "In one way, my heart was being ripped in half but in another way, I couldn't be prouder of who he was."

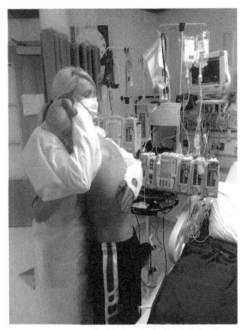

Austin and his mom in the hospital.

Stacy says she can see the hope and fire with which Austin lived in their family's own version of winning the day – by grieving without giving up. "We know Austin wouldn't want us to be in a deep, dark hole," she says. "He was a lover of life. He was so full of life. Our son would want us, along with his brother Cody and sister Haley, to keep winning the day."

Now, I'm not big on superstitions, but I was floored when I heard that the anniversary of Jimmy V's death, April 28, was 22 years to the day when Austin passed. And 22 was Austin's number in football, basketball, and baseball. Even now, Patrick McCaffery honors his late friend by wearing No. 22 for his father's Iowa Hawkeyes.

"When you lose a child, you want them to be remembered," Fran McCaffery tells me. "I remember the day before Austin passed, Craig asked Patrick if he wanted to go in his room and talk – just the two of them. I'm sure Patrick wears that conversation, that moment on his heart always."

No. 22 will undoubtedly be remembered. And I must say: My man Jimmy V and Austin were cut from the same cloth. Jimmy V

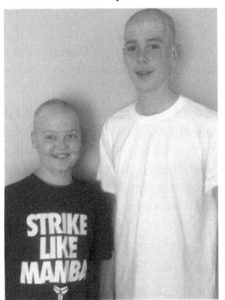

Austin with Patrick McCaffery in Iowa.

keeps inspiring us, and Austin does the same. "They're both heroes continuously making an impact on others even though they're not here," Craig says. "There was a ripple effect to their individual fight."

And it's on people like myself, I believe, to drive their message forward.

Austin's death also came on National Superhero Day. How fitting for a kid nicknamed Flash.

"When you give kids with cancer, or parents fighting alongside them, the gift of hope," Stacy says, "it's like a superpower in a fight against cancer."

So is the lesson that Flash taught us: Win the day.

One starfish at a time.

The Ultimate Closer

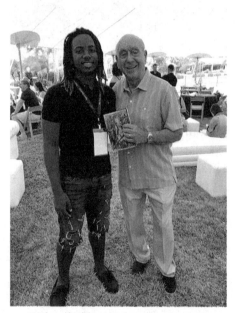

Dick and N'Jhari at the post-gala picnic.

N'Jhari Jackson went into Walgreens to pick up medication for his autoimmune disease. When he bent down to grab something in one of the store's aisles, his leg buckled. He felt paralyzed, which was likely due to the hardware inserted into his leg from a recent osteotomy procedure.

"I was so embarrassed and ashamed," N'Jhari tells me. "A lady and some employees passed by me. I didn't want to ask for help because I'm 21 years old. I shouldn't have to get help just to stand up and walk away."

In that moment, he says, "I wanted to give up." Then he heard Jimmy V's voice – which I've tried to echo countless times – in his head: *Don't Give Up...Don't Ever Give Up!*®

"I remembered what you told me when we first met, and all throughout knowing you," N'Jhari tells me. "You'd always tell me, 'Don't Ever Give Up.'®' In that moment, I thought about our bond, what you've taught me at the galas, what you've been saying in all your speeches, and what you'd say to me when I'd feel low during my cancer fight. It helped me gain the courage to ask an employee to help me up and walk out of the Walgreens."

Wow. N'Jhari's everyday story gives me flashbacks to the night of Jimmy V's hailed speech – when he had Coach K and me walk him up to that stage. Talk about transcending everyday life.

N'Jhari will be the last All-Courageous Team member highlighted in this book. And, fittingly so, he's the ultimate closer. His story serves as a perfect encore to all the uplifting passages you've heard leading up to this. Much like one of my favorite musical artists, Kenny Chesney, it's that encore song you leave the concert singing in your head. You may leave this show playing N'Jhari's story on repeat, let me tell you.

N'Jhari's Jimmy V-esque experience in the Walgreens happened the day before we met to speak for this book. Sadly, it is crippling occurrences like this that can affect cancer survivors in the wake of the war they battled through when they were youngsters. That's especially the case for N'Jhari, who also dealt with autoimmune disease and juvenile arthritis alongside his cancer fight.

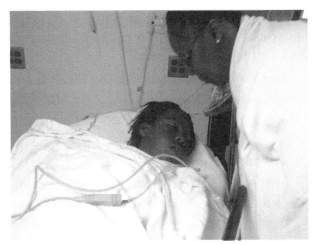

N'Jhari with his mother during his cancer battle.

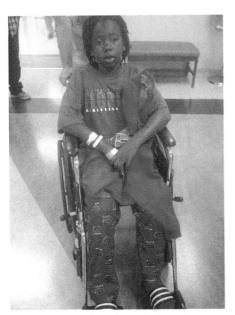

N'Jhari during his cancer battle.

N'Jhari, who was just 9 when he had a cancerous lesion and lymph nodes removed from his elbow, experienced some really great "normal years" as a teenager after he appeared to be clear of cancer at age 12. He starred on his high school football and lacrosse teams before enrolling at the University of Florda, where he planned to play Division I football. But his days of normalcy were short-lived. Residual side effects started to kick in and multiply, and now N'Jhari is feeling the brunt of them.

"You don't ever completely end your cancer battle," N'Jhari's mother, LaShina, reminds me. "You don't just go to an oncologist, you have to have a hematologist, pulmonologist, cardiologist. All these ologists."

LaShina and N'Jhari are a dynamic mother-son duo. But they don't have family in Florida, so they could've easily been alone while navigating serious treatments.

"We try to go to you and Lorraine to help centralize us," LaShina tells me. "It's helped to feel like we have a home base to direct us to different doctors."

N'Jhari has been left immobilized on various occasions and that takes a tremendous mental toll on a 20-something who felt like he was out of the woods and is now experiencing the pains of 50-somethings. It's so unfair.

But that's where hope comes in. The fact that N'Jhari thought of our connection at one of these low moments – when he was stuck, physically and emotionally, at a pharmacy – speaks to the importance of what sharing hope is all about.

Hope to me is really about the belief that there will be a brighter day, for yourself or others. It's the *why* behind not giving up.

> *The thing you have to realize about a cancer fight is that all the treatments in the world don't give you that motivation you need to survive emotionally.*
>
> *- LaShina Jackson*

N'Jhari and his mother can credit me all they want, but I was only passing along the hope that Jimmy V and other courageous cancer battlers have passed on to me. Cancer isn't contagious; hope is.

"The thing you have to realize about a cancer fight is that all the treatments in the world don't give you that motivation you need to survive emotionally," LaShina says. "I don't mean to discredit doctors, physical therapists, or mental health therapists. But I would say the biggest part of N'Jhari's healing process – to this day – is the hope that's come from the galas, from being on the All-Courageous Team, from being around people like you, Dick."

I understand on a more personal level now what LaShina is talking about, being on the other side as a cancer battler. Hope is crucial. It is the one element that's a must for cancer patients everywhere. And, really, for all humans everywhere.

Emily Dickinson's poem of 160-some years ago imagines hope as a bird:

> *'Hope' is the thing with feathers —*
>
> *That perches in the soul —*
>
> *And sings the tune without words —*
>
> *And never stops — at all.*

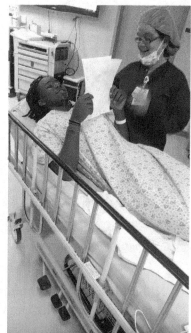

After I finished my radiation treatment this past fall, I was stuck in this godforsaken waiting game. My vocal cords had to heal for doctors to be able to determine if the cancer was all gone and if my voice would be useable again in a way where I could broadcast games for ESPN. Those weeks waiting for a verdict were agonizing. You go through six rigorous weeks of treatment and then have to somehow find patience to see if all the hard work paid off. Are you kidding?

Hope is the only solution in those moments when we feel stuck. Because without it, your thoughts can spiral into worst-case scenarios.

N'Jhari in the hospital.

"Positive thinking isn't something you can just pull out of nowhere," N'Jhari reminds me. "You have to get it from somewhere. When I found out I couldn't play football anymore, I was tempted to go all negative. But I learned from my cancer battle that you gotta have hope."

It's wrong that N'Jhari is going through all this now. He deserves to live a life free of hospitals and doctor visits. But I'm inspired by his ability to find hope in spite of all that's in front of him. He tells me one of his favorite quotes comes from Dr. Benjamin S. Carson, the pediatric neurosurgeon who served as the secretary of Housing and Urban Development in the Trump administration: "Happiness comes not by what we get, but what we give."

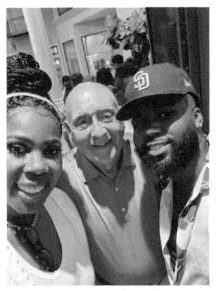

LaShina, Dick, and N'Jhari at the post-gala picnic.

N'Jhari is the definition of a giver, let me tell you.

He and I first met at an event for the Tampa Bay Lightning where he was a Lightning Community Hero as a 10-year-old. We sat at the same table and almost immediately struck up a conversation. He told me he remembered me from the Johns Hopkins All-Children's Hospital when he was going through treatment when Lorraine and I visited.

Even back then, N'Jhari was always thinking of others above himself. He was an adorable boy involved in several organizations such as Boy Scouts of America – and he was even learning to speak Mandarin.

"When he was little, if he heard someone was in need, he'd be quick to say, 'OK, Mom, let's go help.' It was like he just wanted to see them smile," LaShina says.

That was a trend that began far before I knew him, too. When he was 5 years old, N'Jhari clutched onto a stuffed version of "Clifford the Big Red Dog" given to him by a nurse as he went in for a scary surgery. When he was released from the hospital shortly after, N'Jhari noticed another scared kid his age who had just been admitted and who couldn't have any family around him due to his condition. My man N'Jhari was quick to give away his prized possession.

That was the genesis of N'Jhari's "Pajama Buddies" project. He goes to hospitals and gives children stuffed animals, video games, and gift bags.

"Just to see some of these kids feeling so down and then to uplift their spirits in any way you can, it's about giving them that little sense of hope and feeling that they're not alone," N'Jhari says.

He's written four children's books on what it's like to battle cancer, all of them aimed at fostering hope. One is titled "One Poke, Two Pokes, Three: This is Not a Joke!" It is a depiction of what kids go through when battling adult-size diseases. It chronicles diagnosis, treatment, and all the emotions in between to help foster resilience through laughter and courage.

When he was 16, N'Jhari won a prestigious Congressional Award Bronze Medal, an award that's given to American children by Congress to recognize their "initiative, service, and achievement as young people." He also won Eagle Scout of the Year for his work leading a mission to put AED defibrillators in schools and youth sports facilities.

> *Just to see some of these kids feeling so down and then to uplift their spirits in any way you can, it's about giving them that little sense of hope and feeling that they're not alone.*
>
> *- N'Jhari Jackson*

My man N'Jhari's mission to foster hope marches on. These days he's a graduate of the University of Florida, with his master's in sports management and sports law. He's an in-season intern with the Tampa Bay Buccaneers alongside another All-Courageous kid, Cole Eicher. He's a Coca-Cola Scholar, Foot Locker Scholar, AXA Scholar, NBC Universal Scholar, and Bob Graham Center for Public Service Haskell Scholar.

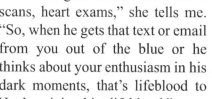

N'Jhari and his mom.

Did I mention he's a Diaper Dandy Scholar, too? N'Jhari is awesome, awesome, awesome, baby – with all that giving and achieving in the face of tremendous mental and physical anguish.

"I'm getting muscle soreness and can't perform the way I used to," N'Jhari says. "As I'm getting older, the aftermath of what I went through as a kid is catching up to me. I'm just trying to get back to the basics like walking, running, going to the store."

LaShina reminds me that the emotional boosts can often fuel the physical ones. "He gets down on himself when he has to keep doing bloodwork, bone scans, heart exams," she tells me. "So, when he gets that text or email from you out of the blue or he thinks about your enthusiasm in his dark moments, that's lifeblood to me. I can't give him that. You're giving him lifeblood."

Lifeblood. Wow. It's special to me because N'Jhari gives me what I need most, what we all need most.

Hope.

Hey, when you focus on the one, you never know if one day you will be the one lifted up.

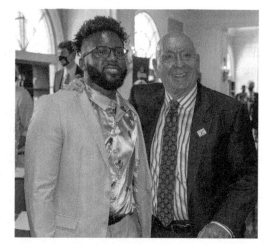

N'Jhari and Dick at his gala.

To donate to the V Foundation,
Dick Vitale Pediatric Cancer Research Fund,
please scan this code.

Chapter Fifteen

Family Over Cancer

with the Dick Vitale Family

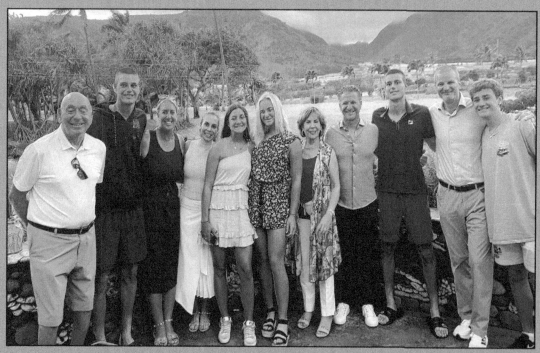

"I've seen a lot of cancer patients, and there is no question you had one of the best armies of supporters with your family that I've ever seen."
- Dr. Richard Brown, Dick's oncologist during his 2021-22 battle with lymphoma.

L ife is all about perspective.

I know this because I'll never forget the best early Christmas present I ever received in the form of a phone call. It was 6:30 a.m. on a Thursday in the fall of 2021. I was hours away from a robotic surgical procedure to treat bile-duct cancer.

"At that point, with the bile-duct diagnosis, there was no clear pathway for your treatment – with multiple approaches, including surgery," my daughter Terri recalls. "The odds were not particularly great. A lot of the family was shutting down when we first found out because it was so overwhelming."

Thank God my gastroenterologist, Dr. Stephen Kucera, called me to tell me a re-examination of my CAT scan at Moffitt Cancer Center, in Tampa, determined that I *didn't* have bile-duct cancer as originally diagnosed. That same day, a panel of doctors at Moffitt concluded that I actually had lymphoma, which has around a 90 percent cure rate.

If I didn't get that phone call, I would've gone into surgery for the wrong type of cancer only hours later. It was that close.

Never in a million years did I think we'd be celebrating a lymphoma diagnosis.

- Lorraine Vitale

"Never in a million years did I think we'd be celebrating a lymphoma diagnosis," Lorraine says.

Yet here we were, out for a family dinner with my daughters and grandchildren to celebrate the bile-duct cancer that never was. You see, it's all about perspective.

"No one would usually see lymphoma as good news, but when up against bile-duct cancer, it's great

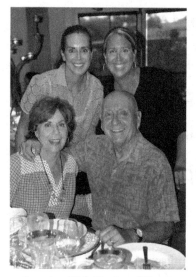

Lorraine, Dick, Terri, and Sherri.

news," my daughter Sherri says. "I remember the moment the doctor wheeled you in behind the curtains and said they found something, that it was (bile-duct) cancer. My head was spinning. You're hearing a bunch of terms for the first time and all these decisions that have to be made in a short amount of time – like who is the best doctor, which hospital to get treatment at, everything. That changed diagnosis removed that burden for our family."

Indeed. The lymphoma diagnosis, in contrast, meant a lot of positive things. Mainly, it was more treatable with a clearcut plan that was universally agreed upon by doctors – with your standard chemotherapy and no surgeries. I was also able to stay nearby in Sarasota and leverage the support of my family.

"It was full speed ahead from there," Terri says. "We were in it together."

Together as a family.

In all three of my cancer battles, if I had to summarize the approach into one theme, I'd undoubtedly go with: *Family over everything.* Family has been and always will be my top priority in life – over everything. Throughout this book, the sheer togetherness behind some of these inspiring families has been a commonality to taking on cancer at full strength.

My battle was no different. I have always tried to be there for my family – and when I needed them most, they were there for me.

My Family as My Rock

When Terri and Sherri were playing tennis at Notre Dame back in the 1990s, Lorraine and I visited for a weekend when the Fighting Irish played Tennessee in football. We went to their tennis match to see the girls compete. Afterward, though, a newspaper headline said something to the tune of, "Dick Vitale on campus, watches daughters." Both girls called me pissed off. They had a fair point – that my being there distracted from the team as the main focus, and from their higher-ranked teammates.

At that stage of my career, I couldn't go to campus without getting mobbed by fans. My daughters, like their mother, are not about the spotlight like me. I love how selfless they all are.

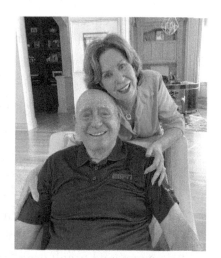

Lorraine and Dick.

132

I agreed not to go to another match, as much as I wanted to see them compete. Determined to be involved still in my girls' tennis careers, I got to know the person at the front desk of the athletics building. I'd call this person during matches and have him relay – over the phone – how my daughters were doing. This was before the Internet and streaming, which is how I follow my grandkids' tennis matches now.

"You would travel three-to-four times a week to cover college basketball games when we were growing up, but it always felt like you were there for us when it counted emotionally," Terri says.

"We always, always felt your love," Sherri says. "We were never left guessing about what your emotions were. If you were mad, sad, or happy, we'd know about it. Letting out emotions is part of your DNA and we got to experience it in a great way with you as a father."

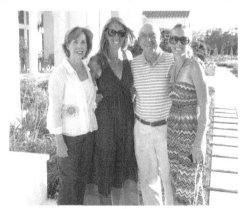

Lorraine, Sherri, Dick, and Terri.

It's true. I love my family more than words can describe. That's probably to a fault because I worry so much about all of them. I've never been shy in showing them, either, but sometimes I wish I wasn't so emotional. I cry so damn easily.

Then again, that love for them is undoubtedly what has guided me in my fight against pediatric cancer. I couldn't love the All-Courageous kids and their families the way I do – because, trust me, there's no better word to use than "love" – if I don't love my own family as much as I do.

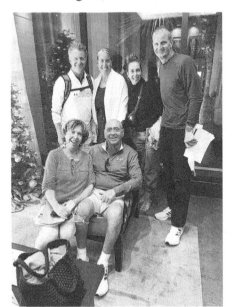

The "Vitale Triangle." Terri and Sherri with their husbands Chris and Thomas.

It's why we live within driving distance of my daughters, why we've created what can only be described as "The Vitale Triangle" in Lakewood Ranch, Florida. Both my daughters and their families live minutes away, with Lorraine and me located in the middle. Terri's husband, Chris, is a surgeon and former Notre Dame lacrosse player. Sherri's husband, Thomas, is a judge and former Irish quarterback. Our three families are always getting together to watch my grandchildren play sports or to debate about anything from politics to LeBron versus Jordan at the dinner table.

The camaraderie we developed has surely spilled over as a key ingredient in my cancer fights. It's firmly made family my first line of defense. And if Lorraine and I are generals in that defense, Terri and Sherri are undoubtedly the best lieutenants to have fighting by our side.

"I've seen a lot of cancer patients, and there is no question you had one of the best armies of supporters with your family that I've ever seen," says Dr. Richard Brown, my oncologist during my 2021-22 battle with lymphoma.

As soon as we had the proper diagnosis of lymphoma back then, it was time to go into battle mode.

> *I've seen a lot of cancer patients, and there is no question you had one of the best armies of supporters with your family that I've ever seen.*
>
> *- Dr. Richard Brown*

"I remember you wanted things done as quickly as possible," Dr. Brown says. "Once we got going, your attitude was that whenever you'd start to feel sorry for yourself, you'd redirect to think about all the kids out there who may have to go through what you were going through."

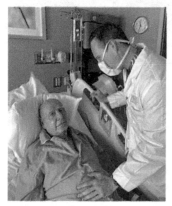

Dick in his cancer fight.

Dr. Brown put me under a fairly intense round of chemotherapy, with six cycles from November of 2021 to April of 2022. I remember feeling exhausted regularly not just from the chemo, but the knifing bone pain that came with the Neupogen shots meant to offset infection. I was also on steroids as part of the treatment, but Dr. Brown and I later agreed I didn't need to be revved up any more than I normally am.

"You weren't the youngest person in the world when we started your chemo, so there was some risk involved," Dr. Brown says. "Ultimately, you didn't just do good with your treatment, you did great."

That's a full credit to my family, Doc. They were my bedrock from Day One.

I felt them carrying me every step of the way before ringing the bell to signal I was cancer-free in April.

Our family strength starts, and ends, with Lorraine.

"You have easily one of the best marriages I've ever seen," says Dr. Steven Zeitels, my vocal-cord specialist. "(Lorraine) understands you and manages all your emotions so well – because she's so in love with you. She may be the silent partner, but you both run the gauntlet together."

I couldn't have said it better, Dr. Z.

My parents always taught me to chase my dreams and shoot for the stars. Well, that's likely what gave me the courage – and persistence – to ask Lorraine out on a date.

"You asked me to dance three times before I finally said yes," she says.

What can I say? Besides the fact that we've been dancing ever since. Last summer, we celebrated our 52nd wedding anniversary.

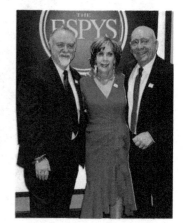

Doctor Zeitels with Lorraine and Dick at the ESPYs.

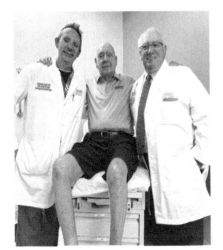

Dick with Doctor Ken Meredith (left) and Doctor Brown.

"Growing up, you really took Mom and Dad's words to heart and grew impervious to people telling you that you couldn't do things," says my younger sister, Terry. "You'd always go for the prettiest girl in school and it never occurred to you that you weren't much of a looker. I remember one time you came and said, 'I've got to go out tonight, can you teach me how to dance real fast?' I said, 'In 20 minutes? And you have no rhythm?' But you'd always find a way how."

Terry's right about one thing. I had no problem taking on the underdog status.

Now, listen: I respect No. 16 NCAA Tournament seeds upsetting top seeds, like University of Maryland, Baltimore County (UMBC) versus Virginia in 2018 and Fairleigh Dickinson versus Purdue in 2023. But the real glass slipper belongs to me, baby! As far as I am concerned, me dancing with Lorraine is the greatest upset in history.

"In some ways, you're like the odd couple because of how different you are," Sherri says. "She doesn't want one ounce of glory or spotlight. She's like the polar opposite, but at the same time, the perfect complement to you, Dad."

"Outward facing, you might appear to be the lead," Terri says, "but to those of us who know the inner workings, we know Mom's in charge of the whole operation. I look at you two, how you care for each other, and I just think, 'God knew what he was doing when he was putting you together.' You couldn't find a more perfect partner through all this. She's been the quiet rock and the ultimate soldier in this cancer fight."

When it came to taking on cancer again – for a third time, in 2023 – Lorraine was my lightning rod once again. She was my voice when I couldn't speak. She made me rest when I needed it. She offered love and support by the truckload.

"She's sort of the backstory behind all of this," says Dr. Matt Biagioli, my radiation oncologist. "When you first came to see me, you were down and depressed because you were feeling like cancer had come back after you felt like you had just gotten through it.

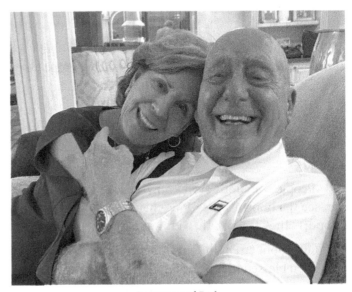

Lorraine and Dick.

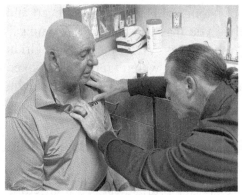

Dick with Dr. Matt Biagioli.

"Whenever you'd start to get upset, she was that positive force to help calm you down and give you the perspective you needed.

"There would be times when I would be speaking to you about your treatment, but my eyes were on Lorraine because I knew she would be the one to police you on resting your voice and lifting you up when you're down on yourself."

So much for me being a co-general, eh? I might have to demote myself because Lorraine is awesome, baby. My entire family is.

As I said at the start of this book, you've gotta have an army to take on cancer. And mine's as good as it gets.

Family of Followers: Public Support Base

When I entered the hospital for one of my first procedures during my battle with lymphoma, the nurses asked if I wanted an alias to protect my identity.

"At that point, you had basically already tweeted out your doctors' names, what hospital you were at, and the room number," Sherri laughs. "We quickly realized with you that there's no regular HIPAA protocol. I think you really thrive on sharing every aspect. That communication basically works as group support."

Hey, I've always been an open book, baby. At least I didn't tweet out my social security number.

"You literally post photos after treatment looking your absolute worst," Terri says. "There's no filter and nothing is off-limits. In a day and age where people take 30 pictures to get the one, you are all about just the one. That's the photo you're posting."

My family jokes about me sharing the raw perspective of a cancer fight with the public to this day, but I must say that the interaction and relationship I have with my social media followers – on Twitter (now known as X), Facebook and Instagram – has been my secret weapon in taking on lymphoma and vocal-cord cancer.

"People who don't even know you are sending you letters and tweets praying for you," Lorraine says. "I can see the boost it gives you when you get down. You realize you can fight this disease because of all the support. They feel like they know you from TV. It's a serious advantage to have that much support."

Talk about strength in numbers. While I've been blessed with the best family a guy could ask for, I've also been blessed to have different pockets of family, including my family of followers.

"I think you've always had this way about you to make others feel like you know them," says Jay Bilas, my ESPN colleague and close friend. "For you to face your cancer battle so publicly, to bring us into your private life, is so uplifting and I don't know anyone else who could do that and have it turn into a strength instead of a burden. You've given the masses comfort and solace all the while you're going through hell. By bringing everybody in, you're expertly illuminating that cancer is not something any of us should have to go through alone.

> *By bringing everybody in, you're expertly illuminating that cancer is not something any of us should have to go through alone.*
>
> *- Jay Bilas*

"In return, all we want to do is let you know we love you and support you."

Oh, I feel that support. And then some. Some would say these folks are strangers. I've never felt that way, whether it was announcing on ESPN or chatting with someone on the street. They're friends. They're family.

My son-in-law Thomas gets it: "Ever since I've known you, Dick, you've always cared about the human side. If someone gave you the choice of eating filet mignon at a nice restaurant with the President of the United States or eating at a dive burger spot with three regular people talking shop, you'd choose the latter."

What can I say? I think I've always been this way – well before the age of social media. The fact is: I just love people. Whenever I see people when I'm out to dinner, I will never turn down a conversation or autograph. Never. When I used to have fans come up to me at the airport, I'd ask them their name and send them a bunch of memorabilia in the mail.

"You've always struck me as an expert on being open and just really understanding people," says Chris, my other son-in-law. My daughters picked two PTPers as husbands, let me tell you. "You're a real student of expression – how people express themselves, react, how they have wants and needs. You have this ability to read people in a minute. Whenever someone is off their A-game, you notice and check in on them. It comes from a grassroots perspective so people can really take to that and resonate with it."

Growing up in a loving Italian household, this is what my parents taught me. We'd always have friends coming over for dinner, passing in and out to the point where my father would jokingly refer to it as a "hotel." My grandmother lived down the street and family was always coming over, having 17 to 20 people at the table. Everyone got a plate of my mother's ravioli.

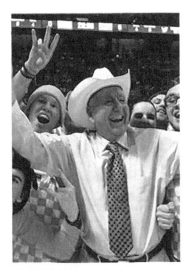

Dick with Tennessee hoops fans.

"You learned from our Mom and Dad to always give back to others and you've stayed that way throughout your life," my brother John says. "If someone wants an autograph and doesn't have a pen, you're the one going to find a pen."

In fighting cancer, inviting the public to my dinner table – through social media photos, of course – has paid off for me in spades because of the tremendous wave of messages of support that I've gotten. The two phases where I had no voice – for three months in 2022 and four months in 2023 – social media connection was a godsend because it kept me connected to the public, to the outside world.

"It wasn't ideal not being able to speak," Sherri says, "but having the ability to communicate with people and stay connected that way has felt like a lifeline. It's why you've always loved your job. You were connecting with people.

My College Hoops Family

I've announced many memorable college basketball games over the course of my career. I've been doing this since ESPN's inception. My first time sitting courtside for the network came in December of 1979, when I covered a 90-77 win for DePaul over Wisconsin. Since then, I've seen it all.

There was Michael Jordan versus Ralph Sampson when North Carolina clipped Virginia in 1983. There was the 1996 Big East Final between Ray Allen's UConn Huskies and Allen Iverson's Georgetown Hoyas. And Christian Watford's game-winning shot to lift Indiana over Kentucky in 2011.

Of course, I can't forget those Tobacco Road rivalry wars of Duke versus North Carolina. The best of those had to be a 1995 clash when heavily favored UNC prevailed over an underdog Duke squad playing without Coach K, who was recovering from a serious back injury. The Blue Devils fell just short in that game despite a heroic shot from Jeff Capel that forced double overtime. Hey, I'm still sweating from those days of an un-airconditioned Cameron Indoor Stadium.

While there have been plenty of buzzer-beating, court-storming games, one of the most special in my broadcasting heart came in 2021 when I returned to ESPN for No. 1 Gonzaga vs. No. 2 UCLA in Las Vegas. My wave of emotions was less about the actual game and more about my sense of gratefulness at being there.

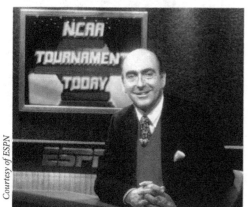

Courtesy of ESPN

Dick in the early days, on set at ESPN.

After the lymphoma diagnosis a few months earlier, I started thinking, "The party's about to be over." The doorways to these sanctuaries – arenas around the country that had given me so much emotional stability over the years – seemed as if they would never open for me again.

So, when I was sitting in a place I call home – on television, speaking to my ESPN audience of viewers – I cried, of course. Calling the game alongside Dave O'Brien, I said then: "I can't believe I'm sitting here. This is a really big thrill for me. I want to thank all of you people sending me so many great messages. … I want to thank my family and all the fans. My, you've been unbelievable."

At that stage, amidst my cancer battle and active chemotherapy treatments, I wouldn't have wanted to be anywhere else than sitting courtside with my second family. Returning to college hoops was the best medicine I could ever ask for.

"In all my years of dealing with cancer, the people who respond best to treatments are those who continue living their everyday lives," Dr. Brown tells me. "For you, Dick, everyday life might be different than others because of your broadcast career, but you were a perfect example of this."

Doc Brown – not the one from *Back to the Future,* but my oncologist – helped construct my chemo appointment schedule in a way where I could still call games that season.

"I remember going with you to a North Carolina-Michigan game in the middle of your treatment and witnessing the enthusiasm the college students had when they saw you," Dr. Brown says. (He is a Michigan fan, so that wasn't his favorite day). "The way you responded to them, if it wasn't evident before, the love was going in both directions and there was a mutual payoff."

ESPN, under the superb leadership of president Jimmy Pitaro, truly had my back in getting me to my home-away-from-home sitting courtside.

"When you came back, it was emotional for everybody," Jay Bilas says. "It clearly means so much for you, but we're not doing you any favors by putting you on the air. In many ways, we need you as much as you need us."

It's a symbiotic relationship in that way. I can't say enough about how supportive all of my ESPN colleagues have been for my overall morale during my cancer battles, from the constant uplifting texts to house visits to check-ins. My colleagues all signed a basketball for me and sent it following my radiation treatment in 2023. When people ask me why I never left for another network and stayed loyal to ESPN for 45 years, that type of support is exactly why. It only validates why my heart has stayed true. ESPN's not just a company I work for; it's family, too.

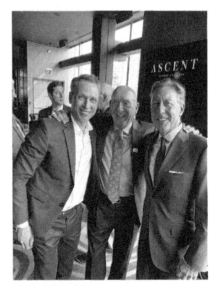

Dick with current ESPN president Jimmy Pitaro and former president George Bodenheimer.

As a former college and NBA coach, I have always had the utmost respect for NCAA coaches and what goes into their profession. I have never swayed away from doing my job – calling it how I see it – but along the way I established some super meaningful relationships with coaches in this sport I so dearly love.

I will never forget when the late Bob Knight – one of my favorite coaches, hands down – got boatloads of letters from other Hall of Fame coaches – including the great John Wooden – to plead my case to the Naismith Hall of Fame in 2008 (I got in, by the way). Ever since then, I've known the coaches in this sport have had my back – and then some.

My bond with coaches only increased during my time of need. I got immeasurable support from college basketball coaching circles. I was unbelievably touched when coach Rick Barnes sent me daily prayers during my lymphoma cancer fight.

"When you weren't calling games, there was a void felt throughout the entire sport," Barnes tells me. "I was already praying for you every day, Dick, but I felt the good Lord compel me to send the prayers to you so you *knew* we were right there with you. For decades, you've protected our game by loving the players, the atmosphere, the fans and especially us coaches. You've always put out the facts about how hard our job is while stating your opinion. That protected us. When you came down with cancer, we wanted to do the same in return."

In early 2022, I had to shut it down with ESPN because, although my chemo treatments were going according to plan, the dysplasia on my vocal cords had started to become an issue. During that time, Barnes' SEC rival, Kentucky coach John Calipari, paid me a visit at my home. John is a Catholic boy through and through like myself, attending daily Mass. He texted regularly to say he'd been lighting candles or taking communion for me during my fight.

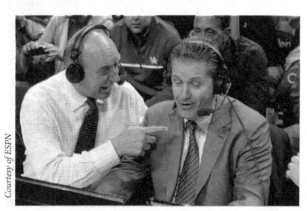

Dick with Coach Calipari.

"When I went to see you, and you couldn't speak, I've never seen someone so frustrated in my life," Calipari says. "We were watching games and I could see you hurting. I was thinking, 'This dude is losing his damn mind because he can't speak.' I came to see you because you've always showed up for me – from the start, before my time at Memphis or Kentucky."

John is right. I even dialed him in the 1990s to tell him his 16 percent interest rate on his mortgage while coaching at UMass was about the dumbest thing I had ever heard. In return, he has always been a straight shooter with me.

"The Lord has been good to you in your life, Dickie V," he says. "If you ever start complaining any different, I'll slap you."

I should slap him back for his No. 2-seeded Wildcats losing to No. 15 Saint Peters in the 2022 NCAA Tournament.

Watching the Big Dance that year miserably from home, ESPN had me filling out boards and engaging in March Madness the best we could, but it wasn't the same. Missing Coach K's last game at Cameron Indoor and sitting at home during the Final Four that year was devastating.

"I remember when we were trying to set a goal of you doing March Madness that year," Dr. Zeitels recalls. "Because of where you were at after resting the vocal cords, it would have been a stretch to call games, but it might have been possible. You looked at me and Lorraine and said, 'I'm less concerned with March Madness and more worried about my gala – raising money for the kids.' Calling games would've jeopardized your ability to speak at the gala.

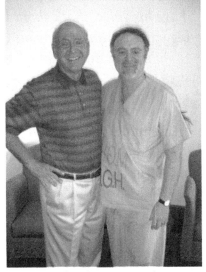

"That was very telling for me. You gave up March Madness for the kids."

Always. If I had to, I would make the same choice again.

While there were many cons to being sidelined for the end of that season, there were some pros. The NCAA Tournament taking place right around the time that I was in my own postseason battle with lymphoma proved to be helpful.

When I rang the bell to be cancer-free, Dr. Brown said, "You're in remission." And, oh my, I was breaking down in tears as if I had just reached the Final Four.

Dick with Doctor Zeitels.

Then, when Dr. Zeitels told me I could soon start talking again, the confetti was in the air and I was cutting down the nets, basking in the joy of winning my own national championship – because I could live and be me with my voice back.

"You hit almost every generation when you're at a game, Dick," says former Villanova coach Jay Wright, a guy who knows a thing or two about winning NCAA championships. "I remember we had a game in 2021 vs. Baylor and we got absolutely blitzed by them. But because Dick Vitale was there, it almost took the sting of the loss away. Our players know it's a big game when you're there. And then our alumni in their 50s and 60s see you as a national treasure when you enter the arena."

I don't know about national treasure, but I do get treated like royalty by the best fans in the business in practically every arena I enter. I didn't get back to crowd surfing in 2022-23 – my first fully healthy season returning to ESPN – but being back on the sidelines regularly provided me with much-needed respite and normalcy.

The season was a victory lap, in a way, and my second time ringing the bell.

I heard the word "cancer" for the first time as a diagnosis just several months prior to that lymphoma battle in the summer of 2021 – when I had to have four procedures to help cure my melanoma. My face was looking like Rocky Balboa after 15 rounds, but after surgery cleaned up the skin cancer near my nose, I was cancer-free. It was brief, but still a short run-in with cancer nonetheless.

> *For a man like you to not have his voice, that's about the biggest punishment anyone can have in this lifetime."*
>
> *- St. John's coach Rick Pitino*

My third time around, with vocal-cord cancer in 2023, the goal of being cancer-free took on a different meaning because, to me, it was so closely associated with getting my voice back. Cancer attacking my voice was as brutal as it could possibly be.

"It was heartbreaking to know you were without your voice again," Jay Bilas says. "Because we know how emotional you can be – and there's no way for this to not impact you emotionally. I didn't want to see you have to go on that emotional roller coaster."

This third fight was exactly that. A roller coaster that felt like it was taking me straight down to hell.

"For a man like you to not have his voice, that's about the biggest punishment anyone can have in this lifetime," says St. John's coach Rick Pitino, a two-time national title winning coach at Kentucky and Louisville. He's gotten three teams to the Final Four, Providence being the other. Let's see if he can make it a fourth with the Red Storm.

"I've been coaching 48 years now and known you since your high school coaching days, Dick," he says. "You've always been at the front of building up our sport when others might try to tear it down. … Your time with no voice had to be total torture, and it probably gave you plenty of time to think and reflect."

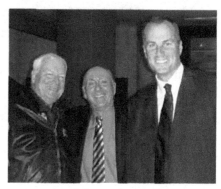

Digger Phelps, Dick, and Jay Bilas.

Rick's right about the reflecting part. As I was stuck in the waiting game during of the 2023-24 season, unsure if and how I'd be on the broadcast sidelines, I went back and looked at the highlight reel of my tapes. I listened to my voice at its peak. I really did kind of create my own vernacular. Some of the sayings in my lexicon are now a part of Americana:

Somebody call up the fire chief to put out the fire!

America, are you serious?

Diaper Dandy!

PTPer!

It's Awesome, baby, with a Capital A!

"Every Sunday we'd have our uncles come over for bagels and coffee," says my brother John. "That's where it all began. They'd take you to games when you were little and you learned to tell it how it is."

"Every time I hear you announcing, your sayings, it brings me back to growing up watching sports in our house," says my sister Terry. "What you say on TV is exactly what you'd actually say in our living room. You don't act any different in person. The difference is, you can connect with all these millions of people like they're your family. You can reach them to tell them about your fight against (pediatric cancer). That's your purpose, Richie."

College basketball has always been my platform to connect with people. But my purpose is to reach people far beyond our sport.

"I was at your house for the first-ever gala, Dick, and witnessed what they've become now," Jay Wright tells me. "When you've come down with cancer, both times (in 2021-22 and 2023), it was shocking to see you affected by the disease you've sworn to fight against. As coaches, we try to inspire and teach about courage. So, I can see so clearly that's what you've been doing – without your voice – by coaching everybody up in this battle against cancer. You've always been a coach at heart."

When you put life purpose up against cancer, we've got a Final Four showdown for the ages. I felt myself cutting down the nets once again one year apart – much like Jay did in 2016 and 2018 – when Dr. Zeitels told me I was cancer-free this past October. For any cancer patient, the relief of hearing those words makes for a magical moment, let me tell you.

To know that I won't be trapped without my voice any longer, and that I'm returning to ESPN for a 45th season to sit courtside, it's truly a slice of heaven for me. And heaven in the fourth quarter – or triple overtime, given my cancer bouts – feels even better than it did in the first.

"If you don't have purpose, you lose reasons – willpower – to live," my sister Terry says. "It's easy to feel invisible. That can't be the case with my brother."

Terry's got a point. That's what cancer wanted me to feel – invisible. Lacking purpose. Joyless. Silenced.

Don't worry, sis. Cancer's not taking my voice, my joy, or my purpose. Not a chance. My *families* – plural – won't allow it.

Family over everything. Family over cancer.

— Dickie V's Cancer Battle Timeline —

June, 2021: Dick begins several facial procedures to remove melanoma, his first brief bout with cancer.

October, 2021: Doctors determine that Dick has lymphoma, which was misdiagnosed as bile-duct cancer in September, for his second cancer diagnosis. Six months of chemotherapy ensue.

December, 2022: Dick is diagnosed with pre-cancerous dysplasia and ulcerous lesions – a separate diagnosis from the lymphoma – prompting him to go on voice rest – for the first time – for three months.

April, 2022: Dick rings the bell and is declared cancer-free from his lymphoma. That same month, he concludes his voice rest with the dysplasia healed.

July, 2023: Dick is diagnosed with laryngeal (vocal-cord) cancer, his third time battling cancer. Six weeks of radiation treatment ensue.

October, 2023: Dick is determined to be cancer-free after his radiation concluded and his voice healed.

Chapter *Sixteen*

My Home Team

with Sydney and Ryan Sforzo; Connor, Jake, and Ava Krug

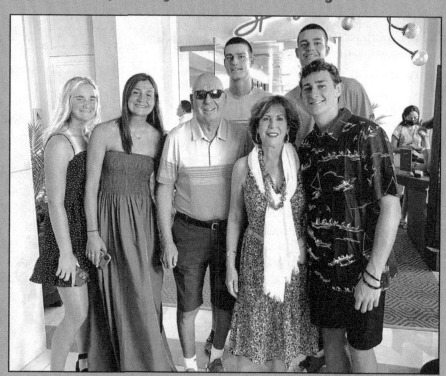

> *"We were right around the same age as the kids battling cancer that you supported. The way you treat them, it's like they're a part of the family."*
> *- Ava Krug, Dick's granddaughter*

I would never be able to make it as a fan at Wimbledon. Not that I would get myself kicked out for yelling at a line judge, like my pal John McEnroe. But it's fair to say that I'm passionate to a fault, and that's why I'd be out of my element in the polite, strawberries-and-cream atmosphere of Wimbledon.

"The U.S. Open is more your speed, Papa," my granddaughter Ava, a tennis star-in-the-making, tells me. She reminds me of a time when I saw her play in a major tournament and couldn't contain myself, cheering at every point. Every gosh-darn point. Apparently, you're not supposed to cheer for unforced errors of an opponent.

"After I won, you stood up and started going nuts and clapping," Ava says. "That's something I'll always remember."

What can I say? Tennis etiquette is not in my DNA, especially when those I love most are playing. I'm as proud a grandfather as you'll find, I promise you that.

Four of my five grandchildren play collegiate tennis, taking from their mothers Terri and Sherri, who starred at Notre Dame in the 1990s. And all that's made me a tennis fanatic, baby!

Sydney, my oldest grandchild, is a senior this year. She plays for the Fighting Irish, like her mom. Twins Connor and Jake are juniors who play for Duke. Ava, my youngest grandchild, is a senior in high school and heading to Duke to join her brothers this coming August. My grandson Ryan is the outlier. He plays lacrosse for the Fighting Irish, like his dad. Last season, as a freshman, he struck gold – like a leprechaun – as his team won the national championship. Talk about an awesome diaper-dandy season!

Dick with Ryan and his parents after the Irish won the National Championship.

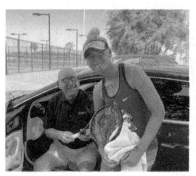

Dick and Ava at the tennis courts.

I've made it a habit to see my grandkids at practices ever since they began playing back home in Lakewood Ranch to today when they're home training during school breaks. I'll rarely miss a practice when I have an opportunity to honk my horn and hail them over for feedback. Just on small things, you know, like moving their feet to open up the court, or perfecting the ball toss on their serves.

I follow every game online. The main reason I don't go watch more of them in person is because, well, it's not worth it to add more pressure to them with my presence. Plus, the anxiety for me watching them is through the roof as it is. I'm sure many parents or grandparents can relate to this. It's just different when it's your kids or grandkids playing. That's why I've always been in awe when I've seen coaches who coach their sons and daughters. Not sure I could handle that.

It's funny, though, because my twin grandsons, Connor and Jake, tell me I'm the patriarch, or "coach" of the family.

"You're an energy giver, not an energy taker, Papa," Connor tells me. "You're undoubtedly the coach of the family, giving us speeches at the dinner table like it's a locker room. You make sure all the players are positioned to be their best at all times. A great coach can manage each player based on what exactly they need in a given moment. For one grandkid, you might be able to scream and challenge him. The other you might have to have more of a sensitive, conversational tone and point out perspective."

Yes, he's right: I challenge Connor, and take a more sensitive approach to Jake.

"Every great coach is there for his players," Jake says. "I can't think of a major time growing up where you weren't there for us. Ever since we were crawling and walking, you were there. You're always doing anything to help us and be a part of our lives."

They're not wrong by any means. I'm always sending them texts, words of encouragement. When the grandkids were little, we'd train in the backyard and do agility drills, the whole nine.

"It was never really even about the sports you were helping us with," Ryan says. "Sports have always been a metaphor for real life to you. You were always the first to ask the hard questions about our play or work ethic, to hold us accountable in a loving way. You were building our character and letting us know: Any success we have, we

> *You're an energy giver, not an energy taker, Papa. You're undoubtedly the coach of the family, giving us speeches at the dinner table like it's a locker room.*
>
> *- Connor Krug, Dick's grandson*

> *I can't think of a major time growing up where you weren't there for us. Ever since we were crawling and walking, you were there. You're always doing anything to help us and be a part of our lives.*
>
> *- Jake Krug, Dick's grandson*

have to work for it and do the dirty work, even if you and Lolo (Lorraine) have laid out the path for us. It's not given to us because we're Dick Vitale's grandkids."

Sports have always been a metaphor for real life to you. You were always the first to ask the hard questions about our play or work ethic, to hold us accountable in a loving way. You were building our character and letting us know: Any success we have, we have to work for it and do the dirty work. … It's not given to us because we're Dick Vitale's grandkids.

- Ryan Sforzo, Dick's grandson

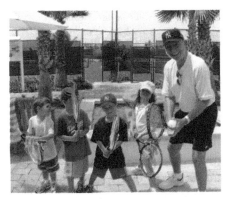
Coaching up the young tennis stars.

Yes, you bet I want to see my grandchildren succeed – the right way. My message to them has been to always be better than you were yesterday. If you don't win, so what? The bottom line is I want you to be able to look yourself in the mirror and say, "I did my best today." They're all where they're at now because they worked their butts off – not just in sports, but academically, too.

I took on a role of mentor and supporter in the best way I could, much as Lorraine and I did with Terri and Sherri before them.

"Now, Papa, it's like a role reversal," Sydney tells me.

I still get emotional thinking about the conversation I had with Sydney when I was first diagnosed with cancer, in 2021. Terri and Sherri had given the other grandkids a heads up before I spoke to them. But with Sydney, she got the news hot-off-the-press from yours truly.

It was one of the hardest conversations I've had when it came to delivering those three terrible words: *I have cancer.*

"I had come home from fall break my sophomore year," Sydney recalls. "I went over to your house and you were sitting on the couch and said, 'Let's talk.' When you told me, I started sobbing. I was super upset. My Mom was crying. Lolo was crying. I just started hugging you. I knew you would get through it, but it was scary because you're older. I debated staying home…"

I wouldn't have let her do that. She's an academic star and athlete at Notre Dame. Some of the best medicine I've had in my cancer battles has been hearing how my grandchildren are doing, how they're thriving. The

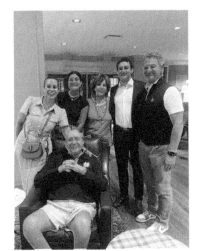
The Sforzo family with Lorraine and Dick.

text messages and voicemails they've received from me during my cancer bouts can attest to it. Their happiness has kept me going.

Still, it was extremely hard on Sydney that first go-round because she was far away at school as I went through my six months of chemotherapy.

"Growing up, you always, always emphasized family," Sydney says. "So it went against my nature to not be by your side when you were going through that."

It's true. We're a tightknit group. All my grandchildren live within walking distance of their cousins, with me and Lorraine just as close.

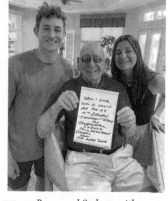

Ryan and Sydney with Dick and his whiteboard.

"The word 'grandfather' doesn't really describe your relationship with us," Connor says. "We have friends where they see their grandfather maybe four times a year. We see you more than that in one week, or even one day. It was like growing up with two sets of parents."

Having all three houses in the same community has created a special family dynamic, let me tell you.

In my latest bout with vocal-cord cancer, the six weeks where I had daily radiation treatment synchronized with my grandkids being home from school. What a blessing. They became my home team to help me rally when I needed them most, joining me for a huge bulk of the radiation treatments.

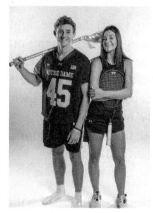

Ryan and Sydney in their ND gear.

It was, as Sydney says, a role reversal. Family has always been my priority and I've always tried to lead that charge. In the thick of my cancer fights, much as with the All-Courageous kids, my grandkids returned the favor in the most heartwarming way imaginable.

> *Going with you to radiation treatments, that's the most I ever bonded with you, Papa. Because it was in a different way than before. This time, we got to take care of you and try to uplift you with what you've taught us.*
>
> *- Sydney Sforzo, Dick's granddaughter*

"Going with you to radiation treatments, that's the most I ever bonded with you, Papa," Sydney tells me. "Because it was in a different way than before. Normally, I'm the one who is more vulnerable and you're pushing and challenging me, you're always good at putting my life in perspective. This time, we got to take care of you and try to uplift you with what you've taught us."

Their support meant so much to me, whether it was taking me to radiation treatments, joining me for breakfast, or going with me to see the Tampa Bay Rays at the ballpark.

"It has been like a flipped script," Jake says. "For my whole life, you've been the one providing and supporting us emotionally. As soon as we found out about your cancer, it was immediately, like, 'We're here to support you, Papa. We're going to get through this together.' You've been constantly trying to help us our whole lives. It's the least we could do."

Sandwiched in between my cancer battles, where I felt as healthy as a young, spry man in his 60s instead of his 80s, I was able to get back to broadcasting for ESPN in 2022-23. That allowed me to call a game at Duke's Cameron Indoor Stadium with Connor and Jake on campus. That was always a goal of mine. It also offered a sense of déjà vu from all my years calling games there when the grandkids were little.

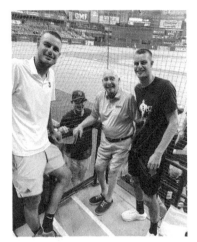

Dick at a Rays game with Connor and Jake.

"Broadcasting college basketball games makes you feel young," Connor says. As I often say, being around the students, the fans, those Cameron Crazies, it shaves 20 years off for me.

"When we were growing up, you were at the height of your fame," Ryan tells me. "You'd take us to Duke games to sit courtside and we'd see you crowd-surfing and we'd be, like, 'There's our Grandpa being a weirdo in the stands.' In a way, that passion was normal for us. You acted this way in real life, too, not just on TV. We'd always wonder, 'Why are people so drawn to our Grandpa?' The older I've gotten, the more I understood: You wear your heart on your sleeve. You truly love humanity, interacting with people, especially kids."

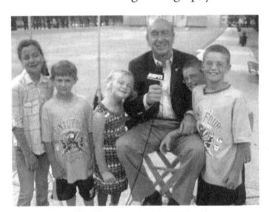

Back in the day...calling games with the grandkids.

"Not only kids battling hardships," Connor adds. "From a genuine perspective, any time you see kids, you try to put a smile on their face. So, when you've seen kids facing adversity with cancer, you feel it. You put yourself in the parents' shoes and it hurts your soul to know they're hurting."

What can I say? My grandkids know me well.

"I grew up going to your galas and knowing about your passion for fighting pediatric cancer just as much as I knew you for your college basketball career," Ava says. "We were right around the same age as the kids battling cancer that you supported. The way you treat them, it's like they're a part of the family. It's not a once-in-a-while communication you have with them. It's all the time."

I've always wanted my grandchildren to see and know what it's like to lend a helping hand to people less fortunate. Life is not as smooth for others and people can have a tough break in life with bumps and bruises. Success is all relative, at the end of the day. Sure, I've been compensated well throughout my life for my work as a broadcaster, but that's not what I want to pass down to my children or grandchildren. I want to pass down to them how I got here. And not just that, I want to pass down to them what I did when I got to the top of the mountain: I helped others up.

Most of all, I've tried to teach them that there's no greater feeling than bringing a smile to a kid's face who is going through something.

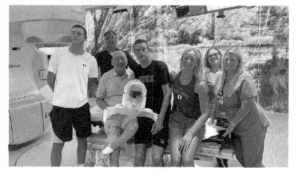

The Krug grandkids at one of Dick's radiation treatments.

"When we went to your (radiation) treatment and the doctors took us back to see you during the radiation – with your mask on – it definitely was not easy seeing you on the table with all the machines around you," Ava tells me. "It really put into perspective for me how difficult it is, not just for you, but for everyone going through something like this with their families."

That right there is exactly what I feel in my heart in this fight. I was feeling it before I had cancer of my own, and now I feel it in an even deeper way.

"I remember picking you up from one of your appointments," Sydney says. "And you said, 'Can you believe kids 5 and 6 years old are doing what I'm doing?' Even in your toughest moments, you're thinking about these kids. If anything, these battles have made you want to fight this fight even more."

You're damn right. Sydney gets me, likely because she has what my grandkids call "the Papa gene." Yes, I've passed that passion overdrive down to my grandchildren.

"They all have some of it," Lorraine says.

Sydney's brother Ryan says he worried – at least at first – that I'd lose my edge when cancer came knocking.

"One of the things we worried about was: With someone with so much life who feels emotions so intensely, would this disease have the ability to suck it out you?" he says. "To your credit, you've used all the love and experience you've gotten from being around the All-Courageous kids. They've taught you so much. It was like God was preparing you all along."

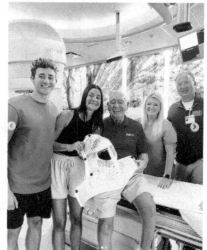

The Sforzo grandkids at one of Dick's radiation treatments.

Yes, as much as my cancer battles have been miserable, I have looked at them as happening for a reason: To show the families of the All-Courageous Team that I'm going to fight. It's my time to live this out. Even in my hardest and darkest moments, I'm going to use the energy and those lessons the kids taught me so others can be inspired.

"You're not preaching anything you don't practice on your own now," Ryan says. "You have every excuse at 84 not to fight but you've always been a fighter, respecting life and trying to make every moment special. You've inspired us as grandkids by doing that, still teaching us. You've shown us that even when your back is against the wall, you're still going to be you. Your story is what keeps us going every day."

Inspiration is contagious in that way, isn't it? Ryan's right about this. Do I have my low moments? You bet I do. How could I not? Cancer took one of the most sacred things in my life with my ability to speak.

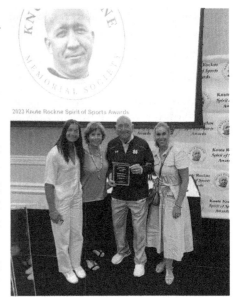

Dick with Sydney, Lorraine, and Terri after receiving an award from Notre Dame.

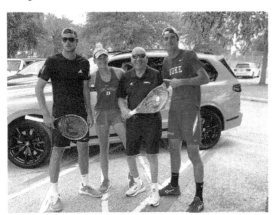

Dick with the Krug grandkids ready to play some tennis.

"Honestly, it was the worst thing that could've happened to you when you lost your voice," Ava says. "We could see how frustrated you'd be with the whiteboard at dinner. You love being able to talk."

But one thing I learned from the great John Wooden is you cannot let what you cannot do interfere with what you can do. And boy, I could still do a lot. Not to mention, I have a healthy family, including my five healthy grandchildren.

"Watching you go through both battles will stay with me," Connor says. "They've been equally difficult, just in different ways. That first one you'd go through brutal chemo and it was like you got hit by a truck. The second one, with your vocal cords, you had to face the fact that you were still at the mercy of the disease every single day."

"I think what's been most impressive and inspiring about your battle has been how you've never let the daunting-ness of what you're facing get in the way of your love for life and family," Jake says. "Seeing you face one of the toughest challenges

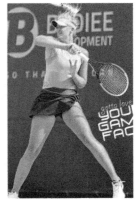

Ava on the court.

someone can face in cancer, always staying positive with your attitude when it'd be easy to get down and depressed, and then say, 'What I'm facing is trivial compared to these kids,' that's a legacy we'll always take with us."

Damn. These grandkids have got me misty-eyed.

Having them be in this pediatric cancer fight *with* me is a gift I cannot even begin to express enough appreciation for. That's because, in reality, they're so much behind the *why* I'm even in the fight.

"Payton Wright was the same age as Sydney before she died," Lorraine reminds me. "Now Sydney's 22. We realize how easily that could've been our grandchildren. I think about that every May for Payton's birthday. If not for the grace of God, all these kids who have had cancer could've been our grandchildren."

Lorraine hit the nail on the head. That is the essence of what's pushing me, why I fight the way I fight and honor Jimmy V the way I honor Jimmy V. It's why these galas exist and why I'll fight – until my last breath, that's a promise – for these cancer-stricken kids. Because they should be living out beautiful lives free of needles and treatment plans, just like my grandkids.

"When some people die, they live forever," Connor says. "These galas and your love for the kids – how they've helped people and will continue to help kids after you're gone, maybe even finding a cure in my lifetime – it's how you can live for us forever."

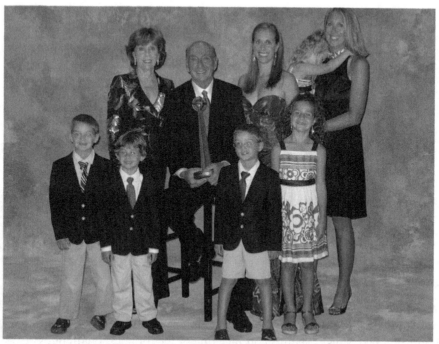

The grandkids at Dick's Hall of Fame induction in 2008.

To donate to the V Foundation,
Dick Vitale Pediatric Cancer Research Fund,
please scan this code.

Outro

A Firestorm Against Cancer

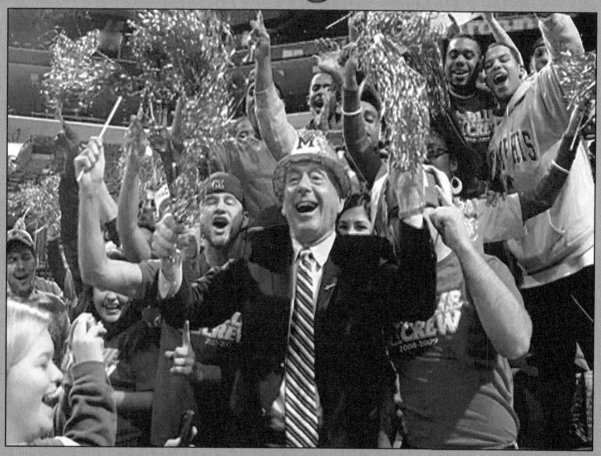

This closing was written in the fall of 2023 after being diagnosed cancer-free a third time.

Remember the Titans?

I sure do. I coached 'em.

No, not the high school football team in the Disney movie. I coached the men's basketball team at the University of Detroit, beginning 50 years ago. We were good, and sometimes great. Our 1976-77 team once won 21 games in a row, including a victory against Marquette, which won the national championship that season.

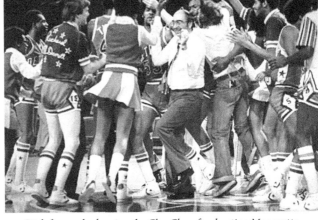

Dick famously dancing the Cha-Cha after beating Marquette.

Not too shabby, right?

These days the school is known as the University of Detroit Mercy. There is one name there that never changes, though.

Titans.

UDM's teams are named for the Titans from Greek mythology. Prometheus was one of them. He stole fire from the Olympian gods. As punishment, Zeus sent Pandora to earth, and she opened a box that unleashed illness and death on mankind.

Those Greeks were really something, weren't they?

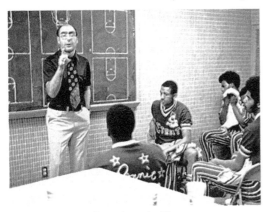

Dick coaching the Titans.

My Titans teams had all-time UDM greats like John Long, Terry Tyler, and Terry Duerod. We went 78-30 in my four seasons there. That's a win percentage of .772, which ain't bad. Even so, you just can't beat my broadcasting gig: I've been calling games for ESPN for 45 years, and I haven't lost one yet. I'm undefeated, baby!

When I began writing this book, I was in the waiting game in my battle against vocal-cord cancer. My voice is my life, and losing it for over four months felt like a curse straight out of Greek myth. (Hey, Echo really does lose her voice in one of those stories.)

In October, Dr. Steven Zeitels ran a scope of my throat – and told me there was no sign of cancer on my vocal cords. Hallelujah, baby! The waterfall of prayers from all of you – family, friends, the college hoops community, my All-Courageous Team, those of you reading these pages – felt truly answered.

Even though my voice wasn't at its best as it healed in the months that followed, my third round with cancer lit a flame in my heart that's only going to keep on burning.

If you have gotten this far in my book, you know I have a set-the-world-on-fire intensity for beating childhood cancer. Prometheus would understand. So would St. Ignatius of Loyola.

Detroit Mercy is a Jesuit school. Ignatius, who founded the Society of Jesus, often exhorted his fellow Jesuits with this command: Ite, inflammate omnia. It is Latin for: "Go, set the world on fire."

Ignatius saw fire not as a destroyer but as a purifier, and he urged us all to go out into the world with the fire of passion and zeal and love. Which is exactly what we all must have in our fight against cancer.

Some people say it is a fight we cannot win. They're wrong. If we keep working and fighting and researching, we are going to get there. We must be, in a word, "promethean."

That word comes to us from the myth of Prometheus – and it means "daringly original and creative." And, oh my, isn't that just what we have to be to defeat cancer once and for all?

We are, in the meantime, like Sisyphus, another figure of Greek myth from the time of the Titans. He twice cheated death and as punishment had to roll a rock up a hill every day for eternity, only to have that rock roll back down and have to start all over again.

Fighting cancer can seem like that. The difference is that we really are going to get to the mountaintop one day. We must keep up the good fight. We must redouble our efforts. We must fight, fight, fight. And then fight some more.

Remember Pandora? She's the one who opened the box that let sickness and death into the world. Here's the part people forget, though. According to her myth, she quickly closed the box, leaving only one thing still inside.

Hope.

Yes, we have hope, my friends.

And with that, we must go forth – and set the world on fire.

To donate to the V Foundation,
Dick Vitale Pediatric Cancer Research Fund,
please scan this code.

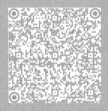

Epilogue

Sunrises Over Sunsets

By Lorraine Vitale

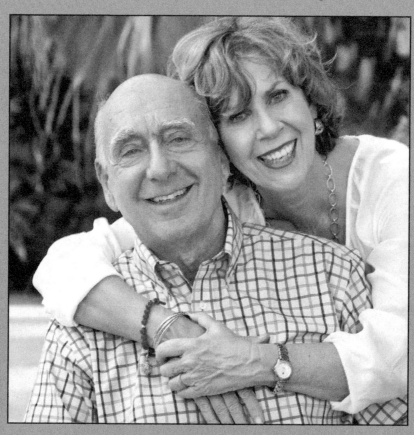

I would wager I have seen my husband cry far more times than any wife in the world over the course of the last five decades.

In 1969, when Dick and I first started dating, men who cried were not considered to be strong. Yet I stand here today having lived a cherished life alongside the strongest man I know.

People who say they know Dick Vitale will tell you he's passionate, emotional. That's no-brainer stuff. Me? I see him as someone who loves his family more than anything – he would take a bullet for all of us if it came to it – and a man who would attempt to climb Mount Everest a dozen times if it meant alleviating the painful cancer battle of one child.

The "Dickie V" persona, the one you see on TV with all the enthusiastic catchphrases, might impress you. But I'm here to tell you that my husband's oversized heart has only been half on display via your screens.

I don't usually hang in the spotlight like Dick. That's his thing. But I know why he has a spotlight hanging over him like a halo. It's not because he's charming. And it's not because he's handsome. Although, both of those were true when he got me to say yes – on the third try – for a dance at the Blue Swan Inn in Rochelle Park, New Jersey, on the same night that New York's Miracle Mets won the World Series. Not many men would persist after two rejections, especially when his coaching buddies from East Rutherford High School bet against his chances of getting me to say yes.

I took the gamble that night on a persistent man who wore his heart on his sleeve. (Did I mention he also had a really nice car – a limelight green 1969 Pontiac Bonneville convertible?) And the rest is history.

It's exactly that can't-hide-his-heart personality that so often centers Dick in the spotlight. In 52 years (and counting) of marriage, his heart has worked like a compass for helping people and making a difference – on a small scale, at first, and now on very large one.

In some ways, it feels as though little has changed. When he was coaching at the University of Detroit, he was handing out flyers at restaurants and parking lots to get people to come out for games. People would laugh when he used to dream big for "standing room only" at Calihan Hall. He proved them – and countless others – wrong. No one is laughing now.

Nowadays, we're doing the same thing with our annual cancer galas. Dick is still handing out flyers for sellout events. Instead of basketball players, now he's formed his own team full of All-Courageous cancer survivors.

Which brings me to this book that he has written amidst a cancer fight of his own. It doesn't surprise me that Dick is putting these brave children out front and telling their stories. Because I've seen him inspired by their grace before, and now during his cancer battles. These children have kept my husband from going to a dark place. And for that, I will be eternally grateful.

I sat next to Dick when he watched a video tribute that the All-Courageous Team put together for him when he was in the middle of six weeks of grueling radiation treatments. He was down in the dumps that day. Then we both sat there and cried together as we soaked in the heartfelt message from all the youngsters in that video. We have come to know them so well.

Look, when you're married to Dick Vitale, tears are contagious. When he cries, which is often, I cry right there with him.

Watching him take in that video was like watching Popeye eat his spinach. Cancer picked on the wrong coach. Because you All-Courageous kids had his back. You are the best safety net any family could ask for.

When Dick told me he was writing a book, my first response was, "What, another one?" He's written 15 books, almost all of them about college basketball. But once he told me he wanted to capture in words – through this book – what has been in his heart most, I thought it was quite fitting. For a man who often finds himself the center of attention, to me that position has never showcased what he's truly about. Dick knows a singer is nothing without his band.

He has always been about the players, the kids, the people who need help. His enthusiasm isn't limited to TV. It's constant. Hey, at least the viewers back home have an off-switch. Dick has always been wired (and, trust me, I know this better than anyone) like an Energizer Bunny – with batteries that don't run out.

That's why watching Dick suffer without a voice was so heartbreaking to see, sort of like watching someone running on low batteries. He was a prisoner in his own body. His voice is his heartbeat.

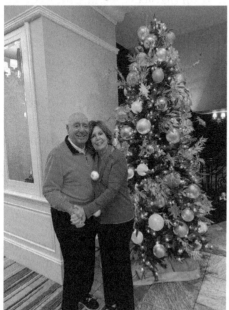

Lorraine and Dick celebrating Christmas, 2023.

Ringing the bell to be cancer-free means the world to Dick, but only because he's seen kids do it before him – and because he knows his bellringing can inspire future kids down the road. It's a mantra of, "I beat it, now you can, too." That is energy that can spread. And cancer is 0-3 versus the Vitales, by the way.

People have often asked me where Dick gets all that energy. I have my answers, but lately I see the answer to a more important question: Why does Dick still go full throttle given everything that life throws at him?

It's because his family won't let him quit.

It's because he plans to be broadcasting until he's 100. (Yes, that's his goal.)

It's because his parents never let him believe in "can't."

It's because the bullies who made fun of his eye growing up fueled the fire that burns inside him.

Mostly, though, it's because of the kids in this book. Kids who need medicines catered specifically to them, who shouldn't have to accept childhood cancer falling behind other cancer research.

Tatum Parker, one of our original All-Courageous Team members, sums it up well: "If his college basketball career were to be completely wiped away tomorrow, his legacy would be about what he's done for other people. What he's done for us kids.

"In that way, it's like he's been given his platform of college basketball for a reason, so he can show the world what's deepest inside his heart."

One thing I cherish about my husband is that he doesn't let fame keep us away from our roots. I grew up in a one-bedroom apartment on University Avenue in the Bronx with my brother and parents. I watched Dick scratch and claw to climb the coaching ladder, and then broadcast ladder. Together, we've never forgotten where we came from. And we have tried to instill that in our daughters and our grandchildren.

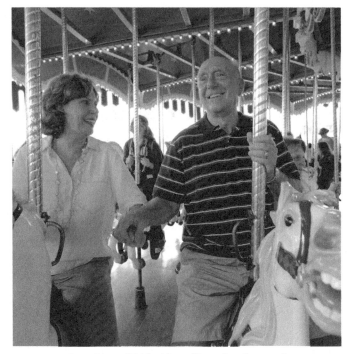

Lorraine and Dick riding off into their "sunrise."

We're not your average retired couple. Coaches tell me, "Instead of walking off into the sunset, Dick just keeps multiplying his ability to reach people."

There will be no sunset for Dick and me to ride off to yet. Not while there's still work to do in this cancer fight. I married a man who is less about the sunsets – and more about the sunrises.

LaShina Jackson, N'Jhari's loving mother, summarized Dick's legacy perfectly. "The love he's pouring into kids – through the galas and All-Courageous Team – that will last long after we're gone and impact my son's kids and their kids. There is no tumor, no cancer that can outrun that love."

Boy, am I glad I didn't say no a third time to that dance with Dickie V.

To donate to the V Foundation, Dick Vitale Pediatric Cancer Research Fund, please scan this code.

Mic Drop

By Kevin Negandhi

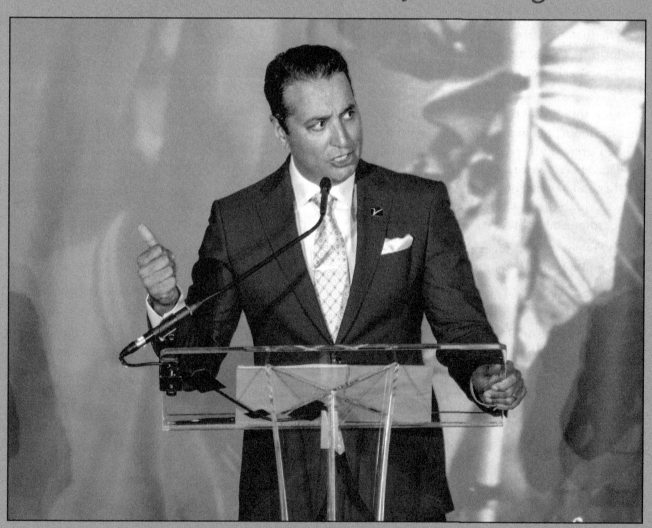

Kevin Negandhi has been the emcee of the Dick Vitale Gala since 2017.

In my job at ESPN, I get to cover and witness incredible moments where stars step up when it is needed most. But for me, there is just one man who is all-deserving of the attention. And, when he's called upon, he delivers every single time.

That man is Dick Vitale.

Every May in a ballroom at the Ritz Carlton in beautiful Sarasota, Florida, Dick delivers a performance that has his crowd laughing, crying, and wanting to run through a wall for him and his All-Courageous Team.

It's in this air-conditioned ballroom where Dick turns into his own PTPer. The 84-year-old Hall of Famer comes up on stage for his scheduled time of 30 minutes and takes over as if he was roaming the sidelines during his days as a coach. A room full of a thousand people suddenly goes quiet and Dick transforms.

Dick takes all that combustible energy from conversation and cocktails and bounces it back like a boomerang to his audience. He cracks a joke about how he had to convince his incredible wife, Lorraine, to dance with him on the first night he met her. More than anything, you get the immediate sense that Dick is speaking straight from the heart. Suddenly, in mere moments, a loud and boisterous crowd is hanging onto every single word Dick has to say. The people are suddenly on a roller-coaster ride of emotions as Dick shares the stories of his All-Courageous Team.

Dick boldly fights for these kids when he's speaking on stage because he knows – intimately – how they've fought to be there alongside him. He knows they've been through hell and back fighting for the chance to do something we all take for granted – enjoying a childhood without fearing long hospital visits or enduring chemo treatments, all while their friends are running carefree at recess.

Dick's attention to detail about every All-Courageous kid's journey, mind you, is unscripted. And when you hear his frustration, his empathy, his plea that more should be done to help young kids and their families dealing with this terrible disease, you fully understand why you're there. It's not to hang out with celebrities, pro athletes or ESPN personalities. It's to join his team in his quest to help in his ultimate fight.

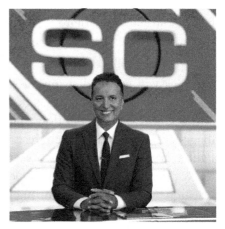

You notice the audience is suddenly in the palm of Dick's hand, ready to do whatever they can to help raise money for pediatric cancer research.

The Dick Vitale Gala's collective organizational group, led by the tireless and talented Mary Kenealy and Janet Allen, and aided by esteemed producers Bill Graf and Rob Lemley, have asked Dick on multiple occasions to be mindful of his own personal health and voice while he passionately opens his heart to the crowd. But 30 minutes be damned, everyone involved in the gala realized a while back that Dick was going to go for as long as he wanted in his speech because, at the end of the day, it's all about the kids. No clock or timer is going to silence Dickie V.

Despite pouring out his heart in a tear-jerking pre-gala press conference – led by longtime friend Josh Krulewitz – just hours before, Dick drives off his All-Courageous Team to morph from subdued to reenergized. His brain is still thinking, "What else can I do? How else can I help? What am I missing?" Dick finds a gear that very few possess and is ignited on this stage when the lights are shining brightest. He shares countless stories about children who have experienced long battles and have never changed their attitude, refusing to back down. He recounts success stories of how the dollars raised have helped in research to save lives and how some are thriving to this day.

Dick also waivers with his voice, shaking in despair about the gut-punching reality of lives that were lost way too soon. And most poignantly, Dick promises everyone in the room that he will not relent.

As emcee of this life-changing event, one theme I have shared on the stage each year since the passing of the late and great John Saunders (who not only emceed the event in the years before me but played a pivotal role in the genesis of Dick's annual gala), it's this truth: Dick Vitale is a Hall of Fame broadcaster, a man synonymous with college basketball's explosion over the last 40-plus years. But he's much more than just a legendary broadcaster. While he's in more than a dozen Hall of Fames, his long-lasting legacy is truly encapsulated in this gala – and through his commitment with Lorraine to helping raise money for pediatric cancer research for the V Foundation.

Anyone who has been in that Sarasota Ballroom in May over the last decade would agree: It's when Dick rises to the challenge and reveals his real strength, carried by his All-Courageous Team, that there's not a dry eye in the room as he walks off the stage.

Dick will get mad at me for saying this, but he is the true MVP of this amazing event. He is the voice for the countless children who are diagnosed with cancer each year. The kids who fight every day and kids who deserve better than the 8 percent that is given for pediatric cancer research. He is their coach through and through.

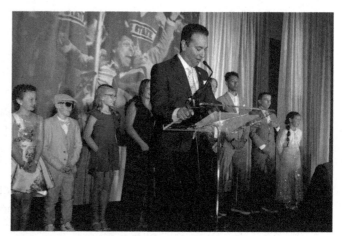

Kevin emceeing the gala.

Every spring, this stage in Sarasota is his national championship and, like any coach, he walks off exhausted and immediately thinks about how he can be better the following year. Renowned coaches who have won multiple national championships are driven off their willpower to win.

Dick has won 18 national championships (and counting) through his galas and that's because he truly believes he *has* to win. For the kids. Dick isn't in this pediatric fight to count his battles won, though. He's here to win the entire war. He won't stop that fight until there's a cure for cancer. That is the legacy of the Dick Vitale Gala.

To donate to the V Foundation,
Dick Vitale Pediatric Cancer Research Fund,
please scan this code.

The Dick Vitale Gala
Through the Years

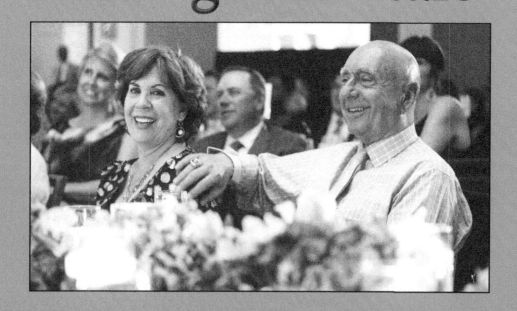

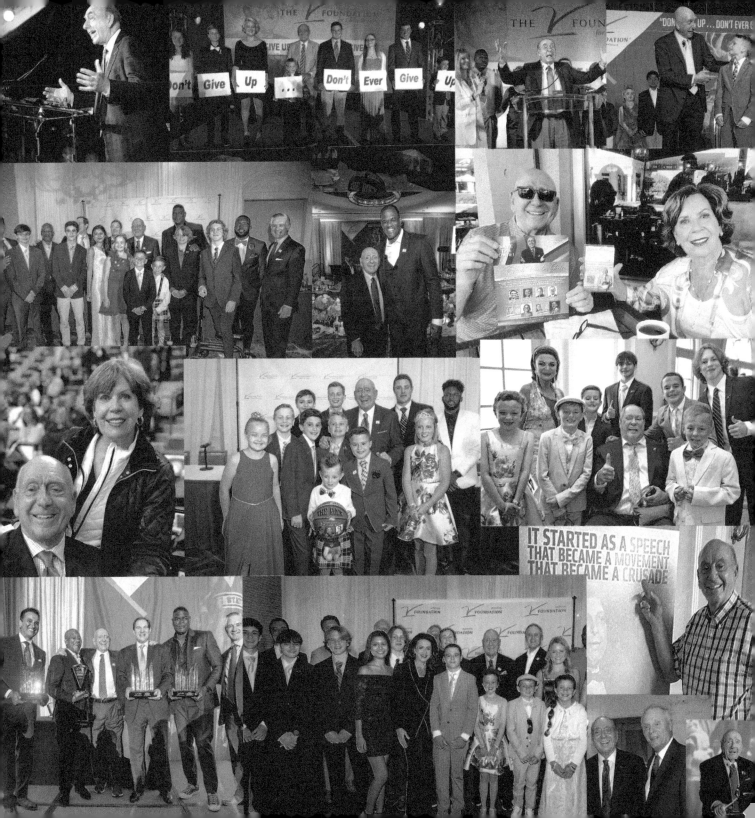

IT STARTED AS A SPEECH
THAT BECAME A MOVEMENT
THAT BECAME A CRUSADE

Afterword

Best Seat in the House

By Scott Gleeson

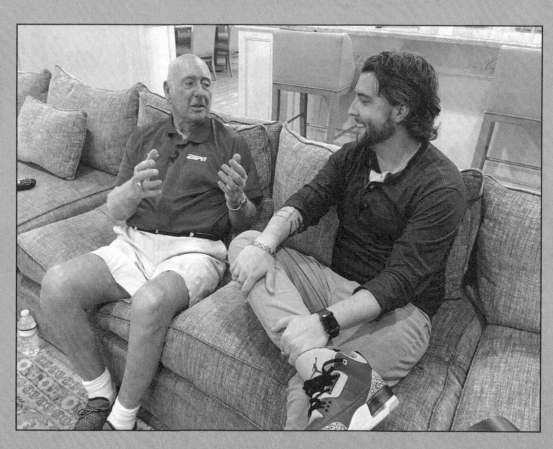

Witnessing Dick Vitale broadcast a college basketball game live is like watching an 84-year-old man transform into a 34-year-old man – for two jampacked hours of bliss.

I would know because that's exactly the 50-year-age gap between Dick and myself.

Dick is hardly someone who needs a Fountain of Youth given how passionate and driven he's wired. But his childlike excitement while sitting courtside and talking to his "friends" on screens back home – with the backdrop of the sport surrounding him – is truly a sight to behold.

The hoopla may seem complimentary to the game from back home, but up close it's of equal value.

The way die-hard fans scream Dick's name when he enters the arena, knowing he's a sports cultural icon to their own generation, their parents' generation and likely even their grandparents' generation, is truly one of a kind.

The way coaches embrace Dick and respect him is even more genuine, with every exchange feeling important – as if he were a prized recruit who could electrify their program.

And the way players nod at each other signifies it's a prime-time game they're about to play in and they just may get an "awesome" or "sensational" reaction to their play from Dick Vitale. Or even garner a "PTPer" or "Diaper Dandy" compliment.

All of this suggests this is a reciprocal relationship between a man who plans to never retire and a sport that feeds off his signature enthusiasm.

But in this timeframe, during the waiting game for Dick's record 45th season calling college basketball games, the feeling is much more weighted to benefit a three-time cancer survivor who was gutted with insistent doubts of whether he'd ever get back to the slice of heaven he calls home in basketball arenas nationwide.

Dick was originally cleared to cover Kentucky vs. Miami (FL) on November 28 of 2023 but had to push back his return because his vocal cords continue to heal from all the soreness from grueling radiation treatments. Despite being cancer free, Dickie V's broadcasting comeback was stalled.

As a sports journalist at USA TODAY who witnessed Dick crowd surf and treat every game as if it were Disneyland, I could sense the frustration that another round of enforced patience was causing Dick.

It's a frustration I saw with my father, a therapist, when his hospice papers meant he couldn't help his patients any longer. Before I ever got to know Dick on a personal level, I knew a man who was wired very similar in how he found tremendous purpose in his career and yearned to help people – until his own last breath.

When I was sent out on assignment to spend time with Dick and Lorraine in March of 2022, I thought I knew who Dick Vitale was from seeing him passionately call games I covered or from all the phone interviews we had over the years, calls that usually started with, "Scott, let me tell you about my gala, you need to have Tom O'Toole (my former editor) run a piece on the kids." Then Dick picked me up at my hotel for this assignment, treated me like a guest of honor my entire trip and spoke from the heart in a way that makes you stop and reassess the man behind all the enthusiasm.

My newspaper assignment was to spend time with Dick in the recovery stages of his 2021-22 battle with cancer, a behind-the-scenes piece. His cancer fight was coming to a close and he had his voice back in limited fashion, but he was unable to broadcast games that March. So here I was watching Sweet 16 games on the couch – in the heart of March Madness – with Dick Vitale to my right. In a story that was about him, a depressed-he's-not-at-the-game Dick asked me about myself and genuinely cared. When the amazing children and families in this book speak about Dick's heart, I can attest that it's palpable when you're in the room with him. But it's also so uniquely directed at you when you're conversing with him.

What I haven't talked to Dick about is why I covered March Madness at USA TODAY for 12 years as I got to know him and why – in its entirety – I felt compelled to join him on this project about fighting cancer alongside these brave children.

That Sweet 16 game at Dick's house was the first time I was watching a game – and not covering it for the newspaper – since I watched Sweet 16 games in the hospital with my father back in 2012.

He died of cancer two weeks later.

I hadn't realized it until a decade later, but the entire time I was writing about Bubble Watch, Bracket Busters and Cinderella stories in USA TODAY's pages every March Madness, I was medicating myself from missing my best friend and my favorite reader.

My Dad and I *loved* watching college basketball. And we *loved* listening to Dick Vitale.

That time watching the game next to Dick was the first time I allowed myself to be brave enough to thaw out and feel my Dad's loss in full.

When my Dad got sick, he wanted to write a book about fighting cancer to inspire others. I even recorded him for a few interviews before his health took a turn for the worse. He watched Jimmy V's video and lived his own version of "Don't Ever Give Up" – living his last 18 months with us as a grateful man when he was given a three-month diagnosis.

One of the things he told me before he passed: "Always follow your heart, kid."

Which brings me to this project that feels utterly serendipitous and deeply purposeful. To say it's been the privilege of a lifetime would be an understatement. But this was a book that required delicate care because of the sensitivity of the topic and all the brave families sharing their heartfelt and inspiring stories alongside Dick.

Writing a book about fighting cancer – and specifically childhood cancer – is often a topic for many families and readers where it hits too close to home. "Thanks, but no thanks" on hearing these rich stories that may cause discomfort could often be the first thought.

That brings me to Dick, a man you should and shouldn't judge by his cover at the same time. There's really no other person in the world, in my opinion, who could author a book about this level of sadness and adversity while finding a way to inspire and uplift in the most heartwarming way imaginable other than Dick Vitale.

When we all watch Dick sit courtside in his 45th season, after being tortured without a voice, it will be like watching a man enter the gates of heaven after spending far too many months powerless in a fiery hell.

But witnessing him fight through that hell to churn out the words and vision for this book speaks to what's deepest in his heart. College basketball may be his career or his passion. But all the "awesome, baby" moments were leading up to his life purpose that's encapsulated in these pages. Dick truly loves these kids and I have no doubt he'll honor the book's title by fighting for them until his last breath.

I found myself believing – whole heartedly – that the best way I could honor my late father, my No. 1 reader who now has his own best seat in the house as I mentioned in his 2012 eulogy, is to partner with Dick on this project. I truly believe that if people can see or even glimpse at what's in Dick's heart, they'll be forever changed.

A question I hear often: "Is Dick Vitale really that enthusiastic in person?" The truth is he's even larger-than-life up close.

This book is a testament to the heart of a man I feel blessed to know.

To Dick and Lorraine: Thank you, from the bottom of my own heart, for trusting me with sharing yours with the world.

To donate to the V Foundation,
Dick Vitale Pediatric Cancer Research Fund,
please scan this code.

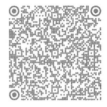

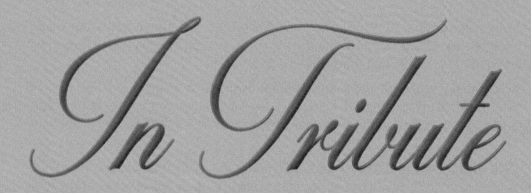

In Tribute

To donate to the V Foundation,
Dick Vitale Pediatric Cancer Research Fund,
please scan this code.

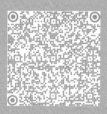

I want to dedicate this book to all of these beautiful young kids who have been to (or their families have been to) my gala over the years. They will be missed, but certainly not forgotten.

- Dick Vitale

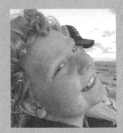

Benjamin Gilkey

December 22, 2007-
February 11, 2017

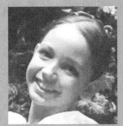

Julia Mounts

October 8, 2002-
April 23, 2016

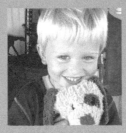

Chad Carr

September 26, 2010-
November 23, 2015

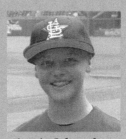

Austin Schroeder

August 13, 1999-
April 28, 2015

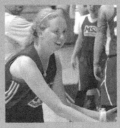

Lauren Hill

October 1, 1995-
April 10, 2015

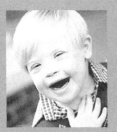

Luke Kelly

January 27, 2010-
January 19, 2015

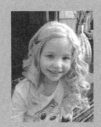

Lacey Holsworth

November 30, 2005-
April 8, 2014

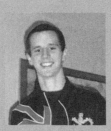

Justin Miller

April 21, 1992-
April 3, 2013

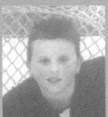

Dillon Simmons

November 2, 1998-
April, 25, 2014

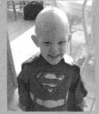

Eddie Livingston

September 3, 2006-
November 24, 2013

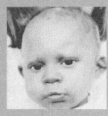

Adrian Littlejohn

February 4, 2010-
May 1, 2011

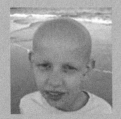

David Heard

May 5, 2000-
February 10, 2011

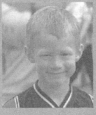

Johnny Teis

August 1, 2002-
April 11, 2011

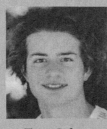

Tony Colton

October 18, 1999-
July 30, 2017

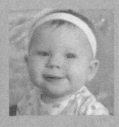

Lucy Weber

June 8, 2009-
November 20, 2010

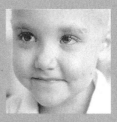

Payton Wright

May 7, 2002-
May 29, 2007

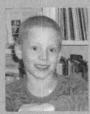

Caleb Jacobbe

February 4, 1998-
May 10, 2006

Acknowledgments

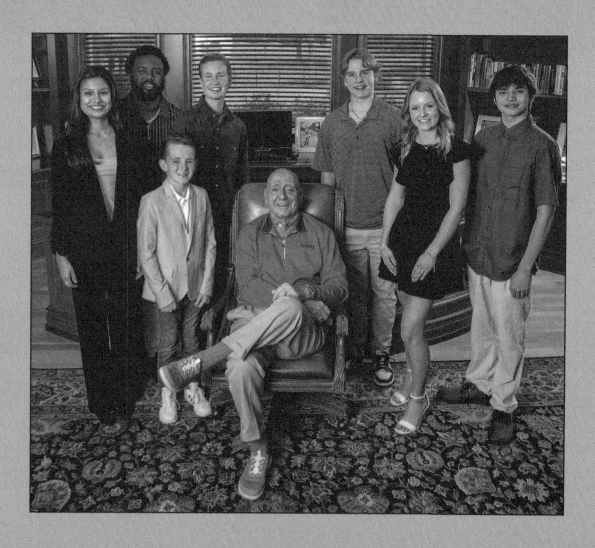

To my All-Courageous Team of cancer surviving kids: You've made me the proudest and most inspired coach on the planet. You are undoubtedly the PTPers of this book. And to the amazing families of these brave children: You're truly Awesome, baby. With a Capital A. To my fantastic wife, Lorraine: Cancer doesn't stand a chance against me when you're by my side. To my entire family: Thank you for loving me and having my back in these cancer fights. To Mary Kenealy and Janet Allen, there is no Dick Vitale Gala or All-Courageous Team without you two and your tireless efforts every year. To Shane Jacobson and everyone supporting me at the V Foundation: You've given me an honorable torch in carrying on Jimmy V's legacy. Thank you, from the bottom of my heart, for trusting me with it. To my ESPN family that has been with me every step of the way: Thank you for keeping me motivated in this cancer fight. There is no Dickie V legacy without ESPN. Finally, thank you to anyone joining me in this fight against the monster that is cancer. I cannot do this alone, and every dollar matters to save children's lives. They are the future!

- **Dick Vitale**

To all of the truly inspiring families who opened up and shared a part of your hearts in emotional interviews for this book: Thank you for trusting Dick and I with your stories. Your courage and strength are the backbone to this book. To my USA TODAY colleagues: You were the best mentors and friends throughout my 12 years with you all. I will always consider it one of the privileges of my life to have written for the nation's newspaper. To the best editor in the business for a project like this, Erik Brady: You've helped shape me into the writer I am today, and always know how to turn a bronze medal story into gold. To my partner, Treslyn: Your love and faith in me throughout this writing journey worked like an oxygen mask when I needed it most. I couldn't have poured into these words without your support. To my impromptu editor, my mother Lynne: I got my love of writing from you, Mom, and it felt full circle to have you read over the early drafts of this book. Thanks for the assist to an alley-oop.

- **Scott Gleeson**

About the Authors

Dick Vitale
with Scott Gleeson

Dick Vitale is a legendary broadcaster who has worked for ESPN for 45 years following his coaching career at the University of Detroit and the Detroit Pistons. Known worldwide for his colorful catchphrases of "Awesome, Baby!" and "Diaper Dandy," Vitale has touched audiences with his memorable enthusiasm. He has also touched us with his passion for raising funds for pediatric cancer research. Vitale is a member of the Naismith Basketball and College Basketball halls of fame. He won a Lifetime Achievement Award Sports Emmy in 2019 and was honored with the Jimmy V Award for Perseverance in 2022. Vitale has authored or co-authored 15 books, including *Vitale* (1988, Simon & Schuster), *Time Out Baby!* (1992, Berkley), and *The Lost Season* (2020, Nico 11 Publishing & Design).

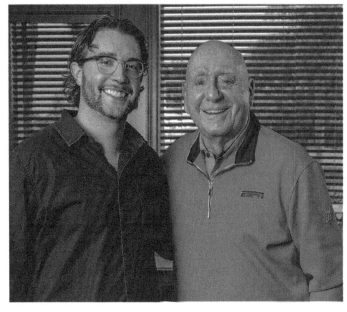

Scott Gleeson is an adjunct professor at Northwestern University. He was a reporter for 12 years at USA TODAY, where he collected writing awards from The Associated Press, International Sports Press, USBWA and NLGJA, including "best national newswriting" in 2022 and "best worldwide color story" in 2015. As a sports journalist, he covered multiple NCAA Tournaments, Final Fours, NBA Drafts, and has been featured as a radio analyst on ESPN, NPR, CBS, and NBC. He's also a licensed clinical professional counselor in Chicago, with a psychology degree from Northwestern.

To donate to the V Foundation,
Dick Vitale Pediatric Cancer Research Fund,
please scan this code.

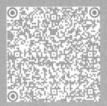

All proceeds from the sales of this and all books by
Dick Vitale published by Nico 11 Publishing are
donated directly by the publisher to the
Dick Vitale Pediatric Cancer Research Fund,
care of the V Foundation.

For more, visit www.dickvitaleonline.com

Made in the USA
Columbia, SC
09 August 2024

40236583R00109